Tarascon Pediatric Outpatient Pocketbook, 1st Edition

The cover is detail from a 1936 lithograph by Mabel Dwight titled "Children's Clinic'" reproduced courtesy of American Artists Group, Inc.

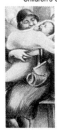

FOR TARASCON BOOKS/SOFTWARE, VISIT **WWW.TARASCON.COM**

- Tarascon Pediatric Outpatient Pocketbook
- Tarascon Pocket Pharmacopoeia® Classic Edition
- Tarascon Pocket Pharmacopoeia® Deluxe Edition
- Tarascon Pocket Pharmacopoeia® PDA software
- Tarascon Primary Care Pocketbook
- Tarascon Pocket Orthopaedica®
- Tarascon Adult Emergency Pocketbook
- Tarascon Pediatric Emergency Pocketbook
- Tarascon Internal Medicine & Critical Care Pocketbook
- How to be a Truly Excellent Junior Medical Student

See faxable order form on last page

"It's not how much you know, it's how fast you can find the answer."®

| **Important Caution Please Read This!** | The information in the *Tarascon Pediatric Outpatient Pocketbook* is compiled from sources believed to be reliable, and exhaustive efforts have been put forth to make |

this book as accurate as possible. *However the accuracy and completeness of this work cannot be guaranteed.* Despite our best efforts this book may contain typographical errors and omissions. The *Tarascon Pediatric Outpatient Pocketbook* is intended as a quick and convenient reminder of information you have already learned elsewhere. The contents are to be used as a guide only, and health care professionals should use sound clinical judgment and individualize patient care. This book is not meant to be a replacement for training, experience, continuing medical education, or studying the latest literature and drug information. This book is sold without warranties of any kind, express or implied, and the publisher and editors disclaim any liability, loss, or damage caused by the contents. *If you do not wish to be bound by the foregoing cautions and conditions, you may return your undamaged and unexpired book to our office for a full refund.*

ISBN 978-1-882742-60-8; 1-882742-60-5. Copyright ©2008, Stephanie D'Augustine, MD & Todd Flosi, MD. Published by Tarascon Publishing®, PO Box 517, Lompoc, California 93438. Printed in the USA. All rights reserved. No portion of this publication may be reproduced or stored in any form or by any means (including electronic, photocopying) without our prior written permission. Tarascon Publishing is a division of Tarascon Inc. *Tarascon Publishing* and *It's not how much you know, it's how fast you can find the answer* are registered trademarks of Tarascon Inc. CY1

Tarascon Pediatric Outpatient Pocketbook, 1st Edition

Stephanie L. D'Augustine, M.D., FAAP
Department of Pediatrics
Ventura County Medical Center, Ventura, California

Todd J. Flosi, M.D., FAAP
Department of Pediatrics
Ventura County Medical Center, Ventura, California

Note from the authors: The *Tarascon Pediatric Outpatient Pocketbook* is intended to be a quick reference guide for clinicians and students practicing outpatient pediatrics. We have attempted to compile relevant clinical information in a concise fashion, and have footnoted relevant clinical practice guidelines from nationally recognized medical associations and journal articles when applicable. Although painstaking efforts have been made to find all errors and omissions, some errors may remain; if you find an error or wish to make a suggestion, please email us at editor@tarascon.com.

↑ : increased / elevated
↓ : decreased / depressed
+ : positive *or* present
- : negative *or* absent
♂: male
♀: female
≥ : greater than or equal to
> : greater than
≤ : less than or equal to
< : less than
Δ : change
AIDS: acquired immunodeficiency syndrome
ANA: antinuclear antibody
BID (or bid): twice daily
BP: blood pressure
CBC: complete blood count
CHF: congestive heart failure
cm: centimeter
CNS: central nervous system
COC: combined oral contraceptive
CPR: cardiopulmonary resuscitation
CRP: c-reactive protein
CT: computed tomography scan
CXR: chest x-ray (radiograph)
d: day
DFA: direct fluorescent antibody
dL: deciliter
ECG: electrocardiogram
Echo: echocardiogram
EEG: electroencephalogram
ENT: otolaryngology
ESR: erythrocyte sedimentation rate
FDA: Federal Drug Administration
FSH: follicle stimulating hormone
FT4: free thyroxine level
FTA-ABS: fluorescent treponemal antibody absorption test
GERD: gastroesophageal reflux disease
g or gm: gram
h or hr(s): hour(s)
hgb: hemoglobin
hct: hematocrit
HIV: human immunodeficiency virus

HPF: high-powered field
HTN: hypertension
Hz: hertz
Ig: immunoglobulin
IM: intramuscular
in: inch
IO: intraosseous
IU: international units
IV: intravenous
Kcal: kilocalorie
Kg: kilogram
L: liter
lb: pound
LH: luteinizing hormone
m: meter
mcg: microgram
mEq: milliequivalent
mg: milligram
min(s): minute(s)
mL: milliliter
mm: millimeter
mmHg: millimeter of mercury
mo(s). : month(s)
MRI: magnetic resonance imaging
NS: normal saline
NSAID: non-steroidal anti-inflammatory drug
PCOS: polycystic ovarian syndrome
PET: positron emission tomography
PO or po: orally
PPD: purified protein derivative
QID (or qid): four times per day
RPR: rapid plasma reagin test
SQ: subcutaneous
STI: sexually transmitted infection
t or tsp: teaspoon
TID (or tid): three times per day
TSH: thyroid stimulating hormone
TST: tuberculin skin test
UA: urinalysis
URI: upper respiratory infection
US: ultrasound
WBC: white blood count
wk(s): week(s)
yr(s): year(s)

MENSTRUAL ABNORMALITIES

Oligomenorrhea (> 6 weeks between periods) *or*
Secondary amenorrhea (no period for > 3-6 months)

< 2 years since menarche

Do pregnancy test.
If negative & no red flags in history/ physical (see differential diagnosis table below), no further workup needed.

>2 years post menarche or change in previously regular cycles

Urine or serum hCG

Negative

▶ Consider thyroid stimulating hormone, free thyroxine (FT4), follicle stimulating hormone (FSH), testosterone, dehydroepiandrosterone sulfate (DHEA-S), cortisol, prolactin, luteinizing hormone (LH). Consider pelvic ultrasound if suspect PCOS or anatomic problem.

Positive

Begin prenatal vitamins & refer for pregnancy counseling/ prenatal care.

DIFFERENTIAL DIAGNOSIS OF OLIGOMENORRHEA

Problem	Signs
Immaturity	< 2 years since onset of menarche.
Stress/ Chronic Illness/ Malnutrition	Identified by history and physical. Until fat ≥ 22% total body weight, patient is unlikely to resume menses.
PCOS	Hirsutism (61%), overweight (35%), acne; ↑LH, ↑DHEA-S, ↑ testosterone. (See section on PCOS page 58)
Adrenal Disease	Acne, odor, hirsutism; ↑ DHEA-S, cortisol, testosterone.
Drugs	Drugs such as risperidone, metoclopramide, isoniazid (INH), H₂ Blockers, tricyclics, opiates may ↑ prolactin, but value usually < 100 ng/ mL.
Pituitary Adenoma	↑prolactin (usually > 250 ng/ mL), galactorrhea, headache, ↓peripheral vision. Best diagnosed with MRI.
Hypothyroidism	↑TSH, ↓FT4; ↓energy, dry skin, constipation.
Androgenic Tumor	Testosterone > 200 ng/ dL, virilization.
Anorexia Nervosa	Underweight, weight loss, excessive exercise.
Ovarian Failure	FSH > 40 mIU/mL; If < 25 years old, check karyotype.

hCG: Human chorionic gonadotropin; MRI: Magnetic Resonance Imaging; PCOS: Polycystic Ovary Syndrome

Primary amenorrhea: Consider bone age & karyotype (see delayed puberty pg. 64)

TREATMENT: ▶ Depends on underlying cause
▶ Secondary amenorrhea: Consider medroxyprogesterone 10 mg PO daily for 5-10 days; if withdrawal bleeding occurs within 2-14 days, patient has normal anatomy and adequate estrogen levels (this clinical test does not pinpoint exact etiology).

Reference: Fleisher. Ludwig Textbook of Pediatric Emergency medicine 4th edition pp 409-413; 2000 Lippincott, Williams, Wilkins.

DYSFUNCTIONAL UTERINE BLEEDING (DUB) / MENORRHAGIA

Normal menstruation: 2-8 days bleeding (20-80 mL blood loss)/ 21-40 day cycle.

Follicular phase: Follicle stimulating hormone (FSH) leads to maturation of follicle and ↑estrogen, which thickens endometrium. Estrogen and luteinizing hormone (LH) surges lead to ovulation.

Luteal phase: Corpus luteum (residual follicle) makes progesterone (stabilizes endometrium) and estrogen. If no conception, corpus luteum involutes, hormone levels drop, and endometrial lining sloughs, resulting in typical menstrual bleeding.

Adolescent DUB: Abnormal endometrial sloughing without structural pathology (as seen later in life). Often result of anovulation in first 3 years after menarche.

Menorrhagia: Prolonged or heavy bleeding at regular intervals.

Metrorrhagia: Uterine bleeding at irregular intervals.

Menometrorrhagia: Prolonged or heavy bleeding occurring at irregular intervals.

Differential Diagnosis

Anovulatory cycles	Endometrial sloughing after prolonged unopposed estrogen. Diagnosis of exclusion, can be stress or exercise induced.
Disorders of coagulation	Von Willebrand's disease, thrombocytopenia, Factor XI deficiency, platelet function defect, renal/liver failure, lupus
Endocrine abnormalities	Hypo or hyperthyroidism Androgen disorders: Polycystic ovarian syndrome (PCOS), non-classic 21-hydroxylase deficiency
Pregnancy related causes	Ectopic pregnancy; spontaneous, threatened, or incomplete abortion; hydatidiform mole
Anatomic abnormality	Retained tampon or intrauterine device, laceration (trauma, rape, abuse), bicornate uterus, transverse septum, polyp
Infections	Sexually transmitted infection (STI)
Breakthrough bleeding	Progestin only contraception, implanted and injectable contraception; recently started new hormonal contraception.

Evaluation

1st assess hemodynamics & determine site of bleeding: Gastrointestinal, urinary tract, uterine, vaginal, cervical (external exam only in virginal girls)	
History	Menstrual, sexual history, medication, systemic symptoms, prior bleeding (epistaxis, dental work, etc.)
Exam	Pelvic exam, sexual maturity rating, dermatologic manifestations of other illness (thin hair, hirsutism, acanthosis nigricans, petechiae, acne), thyroid exam, breasts (for galactorrhea)
Family history	Polycystic ovarian syndrome or bleeding diathesis
Laboratory (before therapy)	Pregnancy test, CBC, erythrocyte sedimentation rate, sexually transmitted infection screening, thyroid, liver and renal function tests, coagulation studies, von Willebrand panel, LH, FSH. Testosterone & dehydroepiandrosterone if suspect PCOS Iron studies if indicated.
Radiology	Pelvic ultrasonography for structural abnormalities or if pregnant.

MANAGEMENT OF DYSFUNCTIONAL UTERINE BLEEDING

Light bleeding & normal hemoglobin (>12 gm/dl)

- 60 mg elemental iron daily, menstrual calendar, re-evaluation.

Moderate bleeding or hemoglobin 10-12 gm/dl

- Combined oral contraceptive (COC, 35 mcg estrogen) q6-12 hours for 24-48 hours or until bleeding stops. Taper to 1 pill daily by day 5. Skip placebo pills and begin new COC packet.
- Allow withdrawal bleeding monthly and continue COC's 3-6 months.
- Consider non-steroidal anti-inflammatory (NSAID) naproxen to reduce flow.
- Begin iron therapy as above.
- *If estrogen contraindicated (hypercoagulable state) use progestin only therapy.*
  Micronized oral progesterone: 200 mg daily for 1st 12 days of month.
  Does not reliably prevent ovulation, therefore not effective birth control.

Severe bleeding or hemoglobin < 9-10 gm/dl   ↑

- *If hemodynamically stable & able to tolerate COC:* Treat as "moderate bleeding".
- *Severe anemia or hemodynamically unstable:* Admit, intravenous fluids +/- blood transfusion.
  - Initiate COC therapy as noted above for "moderate bleeding"
  - Severe nausea, vomiting, or uncontrolled bleeding: Begin IV equine estrogen (*Premarin* = 25 mg every 4-6 hours for up to 6 doses) and anti-emetics.
  - If bleeding does not stop with IV estrogen, consider dilation and curettage.
  - Once bleeding controlled: Begin new packet combination COC. Use continuously, *without* placebo (1st 21d of packet), for 3 months.
  - Allow withdrawal bleeding q3 mos to prevent excessive endometrial build-up.

Management of bleeding secondary to hormonal contraception

1. Increase estrogen content of combined COC's (from 20 mcg to 30-35 mcg daily)
2. Bleeding secondary to progestin only contraception will respond to addition of conjugated estrogen for 5-7 days + non steroidal anti-inflammatory drug. Initially controls active bleeding, but ongoing risk of future spotting.

Management of bleeding secondary to coagulopathy

1. Continuous use of COC *without* placebo (1st 21days of packet) x 3 months. Allow withdrawal bleeding (use of placebo pills) 1 week q3 months.
2. Depot medroxyprogesterone acetate (DMPA), 150 mg intramuscular q12 wks.

Management of anovulatory bleeding. American College of Obstetricians and Gynecologists (ACOG); 2000 Mar. 9 p. (ACOG practice bulletin; no. 14), Obstet Gynecol Clin North Am 2003;30:pp321-335.

CONTRACEPTION

Contraception Options for Teens

Contraceptive Type (% failure rate first year)	Pros	Cons	Other
Male condom (15)	↓ STI's, no hormonal side effects	Need to use correctly	No prescription needed
Female condom (21)	♀ can use if ♂ refuses condom	May be difficult to use	Unclear STI protection
Diaphragm (16-32)	Large dome	Must be comfortable with own genitalia	All must be used with spermicide
Cervical cap (16-32)	Small cap		
Cervical shield (16-32)	Loop aids removal		
Spermicide alone (29)	Woman can use	Messy; possible ↑HIV transmission	No prescription needed.
Medroxyprogesterone (Depo-Provera) (3)	Every 3 month dosing; ↓PID, ovarian/ uterine cancer	Weight gain, spotting, ↓ bone density	↓crises in sickle cell & ↓seizures in epilepsy
Combined oral contraceptives (COC) (8)	Very effective; predictable menses; ↓acne, ↓dysmenorrhea	Weight Δ, irregular bleeding, no STI protection, headache	See section on COC's pg 11. Risk of venous thrombosis.
91 day COC regimen	Menses four times yearly	Possible ↑ random spotting	
Progestin-only pills (8)	If COC contraindicated	Must be taken at same time daily	
Ortho Evra patch (8)	Change weekly, no daily pill	Skin reactions	↑estrogen exposure
Intrauterine device (IUD) (0.1-0.8)	Placed once for long term use	Concerns of increased PID	May avoid in ♀ with multiple partners
Withdrawal method (27)	No supplies needed	Not very effective	

STI: Sexually Transmitted Infection; HIV: Human Immunodeficiency Virus; PID: Pelvic Inflammatory Disease.

Depo-Provera®: 150 mg medroxyprogesterone acetate intramuscularly (IM) or 104 mg/ 0.65 mL subcutaneously every 11 - 13 weeks. Start within 5 days of beginning of menses. Contraindicated if pregnant, undiagnosed vaginal bleeding, breast cancer, thromboembolic disease, liver disease, allergy to any injection components.

▶ Abstinence should be discussed as an option when counseling about options.
Reference: World Health Organization www.who.int/reproductivehealth/publications

CONTRACEPTION CONTINUED

Ortho Evra Patch*: 6 mg norelgestromin/ 0.75 mg ethinyl estradiol (EE). Place patch weekly x 3 weeks, 1 week "patch-free" for menses. Exposed to more total estrogen than comparable oral contraceptive. www.orthoevra.com

NuvaRing*: 15 mcg ethinyl estradiol/ 120 mcg of etonogestrel/ day. Leave in place x 3 weeks, then remove. One week off for menses. www.nuvaring.com

*neither protect against sexually transmitted infections

ORAL CONTRACEPTIVES

WHEN TO START NEW PACKET: Usually Sunday after start period. Can start new packet the same day prescribed if (1) high risk that they will fail to start at later date, (2) no contraindications and (3) urine hCG negative (Pregnancy in newly pregnant/urine hCG-negative women will be identified when no withdrawal bleeding occurs with the placebo pills.) If patient had sex in preceding 72 hours, use emergency contraception prior to starting contraception. Use back-up contraception method (barrier) for 1st cycle.

SAFETY PROFILE OF COMBINED ORAL CONTRACEPTIVES†
(may apply to ring & patch as well)

Safe	Generally safe	Not recommended	Contraindicated
•Up to 40 years old •>21 days postpartum & *not* breastfeeding •Post-abortion or ectopic pregnancy •Benign breast disease •Family history of breast cancer* •HIV •Viral hepatitis carrier •Hypo/ hyper-thyroidism •Varicose veins •Minor surgery	•HIV on medications •> 6 months postpartum & breastfeeding •< 35 years old & smoker •Valvular disease (uncomplicated) •Family history DVT/PE •Body Mass Index (BMI) > 30 •Asymptomatic gallbladder disease •Migraine without aura in patient <35 years old •Diabetes, sickle cell disease •Hypertension in pregnancy	•Gallbladder disease •6 weeks-6 months postpartum & breastfeeding •< 21 days postpartum •35 yr old & smokes < 15 cigarettes/day •Rifampin therapy •Some anticonvulsants¥ •History of or well controlled hypertension •Breast cancer in remission > 5 years •On antibiotics •Hyperlipidemia	•Migraine with aura •< 6 weeks postpartum & breastfeeding •Complicated heart disease or diabetes •Blood Pressure > 160/ 100 •History of DVT/PE •Liver disease •Prolonged immobilization, major surgery. •Ischemic heart disease /Stroke •↑ risk thrombosis‡ •Breast cancer

DVT: Deep Venous Thrombosis; HTN: Hypertension; PE: Pulmonary Embolism

*slight ↑ risk with BRCA1 mutation;   ¥carbamazepine, topiramate, barbiturates, phenytoin;
‡ Factor V Leiden, Protein C or S deficiency;   † Medical eligibility criteria for contraceptive use World Health Organization; 2004. www.who.int/reproductive health/publications.

CONTRACEPTION CONTINUED

ORAL CONTRACEPTIVES

Monophasic	Estrogen (mcg)	Progestin (mg)
Norinyl1+50, Ortho novum 1/50, Necon 1/50	50 mestranol	1 norethindrone
Ovcon-50	50 ethinyl estradiol (EE)	
Demulen 1/50, Zovia 1/50E		1 ethynodiol
Ovral, Ogestrel		0.5 norgestrel
Norinyl 1+35, Ortho-Novum1/35, Necon 1/35, Nortrel 1/35	35 ethinyl estradiol (EE)	1 norethindrone
Brevicon, Modicon, Necon/ Nortrel 0.5/35,		0.5 NORE
Ovcon-35		0.4 NORE
Previfem		0.18 NORG
Ortho-Cyclen, MonoNessa, Sprintec-28		0.25 NORG
Demulen 1/35, Zovia 1/35E		1 ethynodiol
Loestrin 21 1.5/30, Loestrin Fe 1.5/30, Junel 1.5/30, Junel 1.5/ 30 Fe, Microgestin Fe 1.5/30	30 ethinyl estradiol (EE)	1.5 NORE
Cryselle, Lo/ Ovral, Low-Ogestrel		0.3 norgestrel
Apri, Desogen, Ortho-Cept		0.15 desogestrel
Levlen, Levora, Nordette, Portia, Seasonale*		0.15 LEVO
Yasmin		3 drospirenone
Loestrin 21 1/20, Loestrin Fe 1/20, Junel 1/20, Junel Fe 1/20, Microgestin Fe 1/20	20 ethinyl estradiol (EE)	1 norethindrone
Alesse, Aviane, Lessina, Levlite		0.1 LEVO
Progestin Only		
Micronor, Nor-Q.D., Camila, Errin, Jolivette, Nora-BE	none	0.35 NOR
Ovrette		0.075 norgestrel
Biphasic (estrogen/ progestin varies)		
Kariva, Mircette	20/10 EE	0.15/0 DES
Ortho Novum 10/11, Necon 10/11	35 EE	0.5/1 NORE
Triphasic (estrogen/ progestin varies)		
Cyclessa, Velivet	25 EE	0.1/0.125/0.15 desogestrel
Ortho-Novum 7/7/7, Necon 7/7/7, Nortrel 7/7/7	35 EE	0.5/0.75/1 NORE
Tri-Norinyl		0.5/1/0.5 NORE
Enpresse, Tri-Levlen, Triphasil, Trivora-28	30/40/30 EE	0.5/0.75/0.125 levonorgestrel
Ortho Tri-Cyclen, Trinessa, Tri-Sprintec, Tri-Previfem	35 EE	0.18/0.215/0.25 norgestimate
Ortho Tri-Cyclen Lo	25 EE	
Estrostep Fe	20/30/35 EE	1 norethindrone

NORE= Norethindrone; DES= Desogestrel; NOR= Norgestrel; NORG= Norgestimate; LEVO=levonorgestrel

CONTRACEPTION CONTINUED

Specific indications for certain oral contraceptives:

Mircette	Menstrual-related migraines (no aura)
Estrostep Fe	Minimizes breakthrough bleeding
Seasonale	4 periods/year (84 pill pack). This concept works with any low dose monophasic combined oral contraceptive: Skip placebo & start new pill pack for 2 consecutive months before using placebo.
Yasmin	Anti-androgen effects. May help with dysmenorrhea, acne, endometriosis, cystic breasts, and anemia related to menses.

MISSED PILLS:
▶ 1-2 pills missed with _no_ sex in past 5 days: Take 2 pills as soon as you remember, continue on with pack, and use backup method for 1 week.
▶ 1-2 pills missed _and_ <u>has had sex</u> in past 5 days: Emergency contraception (see below) then resume pill pack.
▶ > 4 pills missed: Skip the rest of that pill pack and start new one. Use backup method of contraception for one month.

EMERGENCY CONTRACEPTION (EC):
Taking one of the following regimens within 72 hours (possibly 120 hours) after unprotected sex decreases risk of pregnancy by 89-95%.
▶ _Plan B:_ Levonorgestrel 0.75 mg. 1 pill PO now, then 1 pill PO in 12 hours; (both at once is as effective but not FDA approved); ↓ nausea when pills taken 12 hours apart (23% vs 50% for combined method)
▶ _Ogestrel, Ovral:_ 2 white pills now, 2 white pills in 12 hours.
▶ _Cryselle, Levora, Low Ogestrel_ or _Lo/Ovral_ white pills; _Nordette_ or _Levlen_ light orange pills; _Tri-Levlen_ or _Triphasil_ yellow pills; _Seasonale_ or _Trivora_ pink pills: 4 pills now and 4 pills in 12 hours.
▶ _Levlite, Alesse,_ or _Lessina_ pink pills; _Aviane_ orange pills: 5 pills now, repeat in 12 hours
▶ Contraindications for progestin-only emergency contraception: pregnancy, allergy, abnormal vaginal bleeding
▶ Contraindications for combined oral contraceptives: Same as general use of combined oral contraceptives (see pg 10).
▶ More information at www.not-2-late.com or www.managingcontraception.com

Feldman, _Contraceptive Care for the Adolescent_; Primary Care Clinics in Office Practice 33:2 6/06; Conrad/ Gold, Contemporary Pediatrics 23:2 2/06. Table of Oral Contraceptive adapted with permission from Tarascon Pocket Pharmacopoeia 2007

		SEXUALLY TRANSMITTED INFECTIONS - 1		
Organism	Clinical features	Diagnosis	Treatment	Other
Chlamydia trachomatis	Usually asymptomatic. ♀: Discharge, bleeding, pain with sex, urethritis. ♂: dysuria, discharge, epididymitis.	•NAAT: Nucleic acid amplification test (urine or swab) •DFA •Culture DNA probe	Azithromycin 1g PO x1 or Doxycycline 100 mg PO BID x 7 days Or Ofloxacin 300 mg PO BID x 7 days	•NAAT may be positive for 3 weeks after treatment •Screen sexually active yearly •Treat for gonorrhea also. •Report to public health •Test and treat partners
Neisseria gonorrhea	♀: Usually asymptomatic. May have: urethritis, cervicitis, salpingitis, PID, hepatitis, conjunctivitis, or disseminated disease. ♂: Usually symptomatic; dysuria, pyuria, discharge, epididymitis, conjunctivitis.	•Culture •Nucleic acid amplification (urine or swab)	Ceftriaxone 125 mg IM x 1 Or Cefixime 400 mg PO x 1 (200mg/ 5 mL suspension)	•Report to public health. •Test/ treat partners. •Screen yearly. •Consider treating for chlamydia also. •Check HIV test
Herpes simplex virus	Tingling/ burning Dysuria (♀ 83%, ♂ 44%) Discharge Systemic symptoms, especially in primary infection.

Vesicles and pustules. | (sensitivity in parenthesis) •Tzanck smear (30-80%) •PAP (40%) •Culture (25-94% depends on stage) •DNA probe/ PCR (very sensitive; expensive) •Type specific antibodies (serology) | **Primary infection:** Acyclovir 400 mg PO TID x 7-10 days (within 6 days of onset) **Recurrent Infection:** Acyclovir 400 mg PO TID x 5 days or 800 mg PO BID x 5 days; **Daily suppressive therapy** (if > 6 HSV / yr): Acyclovir 400 mg PO BID; **Oral herpes:** Penciclovir cream Q2 hours x 4 d (or PO acyclovir) | •PO acyclovir in primary infection ↓ viral shedding by 10 days, new lesions (40%), pain (25%), time to healing (4-9 days). Treatment does not change recurrence.

•Less studies with famciclovir or valacyclovir.

www. herpes-foundation.org |

SEXUALLY TRANSMITTED INFECTIONS – 2

Organism	Clinical features	Diagnosis	Treatment	Other
Human papilloma virus (HPV) = warts)	Incubation 3 weeks-8 months; 4 types: Condyloma acuminata, papular, keratotic, flat-topped warts. Usually asymptomatic Vaccine: human papilloma virus recombinant vaccine (*Gardasil*) protects vs. 4 types which cause 70% of cervical cancer and 90% of genital warts.	Physical inspection for external genital warts. PAP smear for cervical infection with HPV.	**External warts:** •Imiquimod (*Aldara*) 5% cream: Apply for 6-10 hours then wash off. **OR** •Podofilox 0.5% solution/ gel applied BID x 3 days; may repeat in 4 days if needed. **Internal /External:** •Liquid nitrogen/ cryotherapy (cryoprobe not recommended: Risk of fistula formation.) •Trichloroacetic acid (TCA) or Bichloroacetic acid.	Imiquimod may weaken condoms/ diaphragm; use 3x/week for 16 weeks. Recurrence possible with any treatment. Molluscum contagiosum can also be treated with TCA, podophyllin or liquid nitrogen. www.ashastd.org Topical treatments not recommended in pregnancy.
Pediculosis pubis	Asymptomatic or itching; 1-2 weeks after exposure.	Nits on hair shafts (small, cream colored, oval).	Permethrin 1% x 10 minutes.	May need to repeat in 7 days Eyelash infections treated with ophthalmic ointment.
Chancroid (H ducreyi)	Painful genital ulcer with inguinal adenopathy.	•Culture for H. ducreyi (< 80% sensitive); •PCR (not available everywhere) •Rule out herpes & syphilis	Azithromycin 1 g PO x 1 **OR** Ceftriaxone 250 mg intramuscularly x 1 **OR** Ciprofloxacin 500 mg PO BID x 3 days, **OR** Erythromycin base 500 mg PO TID x 7 days.	10% co-infected with herpes or syphilis. Test for HIV and syphilis now and again in 3 months. Treat partners.

SEXUALLY TRANSMITTED INFECTIONS – 3

Organism	Clinical features	Diagnosis	Treatment	Other
Trichomonas	Foul smelling yellow discharge or no symptoms	Microscopy (60% sensitive) Culture	**Metronidazole** 2 g orally in a single dose	Treat partners. 70% transmission rate.
HIV	Often asymptomatic; may have fever, adenopathy, rash, malaise in first few weeks after infection.	Must obtain consent; Screening: HIV-1 and HIV-2 by EIA. Confirm + screen with western blot or an immunofluorescence assay (IFA). 95% + by 3 months.	Counseling; rule out other STI's; place PPD; viral load; antiretrovirals, vaccines, and prophylaxis for opportunistic infections if indicated.	If acute syndrome & < 3 months from possible infection, may consider HIV RNA (viral load) testing (and confirm with another test if +).
Syphilis	1°: chancre (painless) 2°: rash, adenopathy, mucocutaneous lesions latent: asymptomatic	VDRL &/or RPR+ and FTA-ABS &/or TP-PA + DFA of lesion. Also test for HIV.	**Benzathine penicillin G** 50,000 units/kg IM, up to the adult dose of 2.4 million units (single dose).	Jarisch-Herxheimer reaction: Fever, headache, myalgia 24 hours after treatment initiated.
Bacterial vaginosis	White discharge, or asymptomatic	3 of 4: white discharge, clue cells, vaginal pH >4.5, fish odor with KOH	**Metronidazole** 500 mg PO bid X 7 days, OR **Metronidazole gel** 0.75%, (5 g) vaginally daily X 5 days OR **Clindamycin** cream 2% (5 g) vaginally nightly X 7 days.	Fem Exam® test card & similar cards may be useful diagnostic tests. (www.coopersurgical.com) **Alternate treatment regimen: Metronidazole** 2 g orally in a single dose.
Vulvar / vaginal candidiasis	Discharge, itching, burning	Potassium hydroxide (KOH) + microscopy	**Miconazole** 2% cream 5 g vaginally X 7 days, or **Tioconazole** 6.5% ointment 5 g vaginally X 1	Creams may weaken condoms. **Oral treatment alternative: Fluconazole** 150 mg tablet PO X 1.

SEXUALLY TRANSMITTED INFECTIONS – 4

Organism	Clinical features	Diagnosis	Treatment	Other
PID (gonorrhea, chlamydia, anaerobes, strep, gram negatives)	Fever, discharge, adnexal tenderness, cervical motion tenderness	Cervical motion /adnexal tenderness; ± fever, ↑CRP/ ESR/ WBC, +/- Gonorrhea or chlamydia testing	**Doxycycline** 100 mg PO bid x 14 days + single IM dose ceftriaxone 250 mg (**OR Levofloxacin** 500 mg PO daily ± **Metronidazole** 500 mg PO bid x 14 days)	Hospitalize if: Severe illness, cannot rule out other causes of abdominal pain, vomiting, tubo-ovarian abscess, pregnant, failed outpatient treatment.
Hepatitis B	May be asymptomatic or have abdominal pain, vomiting, jaundice	See chart below.	Supportive care; antivirals for chronic infection. Prophylaxis to sexual contacts within 14 days.	Infection is more likely to become chronic when infected at a younger age.
Hepatitis C	Asymptomatic to liver failure	Anti-HCV antibodies; if + HCV RNA PCR & ALT level.	Consult specialist.	MMWR Recomm Rep - 10-MAY-2002; 51(RR-6): 1-78

SEROLOGY IN HEPATITIS B INFECTION

	HBsAg	Anti-HBs	Anti-HBc	Total Hepatitis B IgM
Acute infection	+	-	+	+
Chronic infection	+	-	+	-
Immunized	-	+	-	-

CRP= C Reactive Protein; ESR= Sedimentation Rate; WBC= White blood cell count; HBsAg= Hepatitis B Surface Antigen; Anti-HBs=Antibodies to Hepatitis B Surface Antigen; Anti-HBc= Antibodies to Hepatitis B Core Antigen; IgM= Immunoglobulin M.
PID= Pelvic inflammatory disease.
Reference: Sexually Transmitted Diseases Treatment Guidelines 2006, Centers for Disease Control and Prevention

MANAGEMENT OF ANAPHYLAXIS

Secure airway, check breathing & circulation. CPR if indicated. Oxygen. Call 911

Administer Medications as indicated by severity of reaction

Epinephrine 1:1000: 0.01 ml/kg (max 0.3 ml) SQ or IM as often as q15 min	
or	
Epinephrine 1:10000: 0.1 ml/kg IV or IO over 1-2 minutes if ↓perfusion	
or	
Pre-filled epinephrine solutions	EpiPen Jr (for patients <30 kg) IM or SQ, or EpiPen (for patients >30 kg) IM or SQ

Histamine-1 (H₁) blocking drugs

Diphenhydramine	1 mg/kg (max 50 mg) PO, IM, or IV
or	
Hydroxyzine	0.5 mg/kg IV or PO (max dose 25 mg)

Glucocorticoids to prevent late-onset inflammation

Methylprednisolone	1-2 mg/kg IV (max dose 125 mg)
or	
Prednisone	1-2 mg/kg PO (max dose 60 mg)

Consider Histamine-2 (H₂) blocker as adjunct to H₁ blockers

Cimetidine	5 mg/kg (max dose 300 mg) PO/IV/IM
or	
Ranitidine	1-2 mg/kg (max dose 50 mg) PO/IV/IM

Nebulized medications for bronchospasm   If hypotensive

Albuterol solutions (q 20 min x 3 as needed) •0.5% (5 mg/ml) = dilute in normal saline to 3 ml •0.083% = 0.83 mg/ml	Dose based on weight <15 kg: 1.25 mg 15-30 kg: 2.5 mg >30 kg: 5 mg
Racemic epinephrine (2.25%): 0.25-0.5 ml (dilute in 2.5 ml normal saline)	

Trendelenburg position
Normal saline bolus (20 ml/kg)

IM: Intramuscular, IO: Intraosseous, IV: Intravenously, NS: Normal saline, PO: orally, SQ: Subcutaneous

URTICARIA (HIVES)

- **Definition**: Transient, superficial swelling caused by localized capillary vasodilation with plasma transudation, in reaction to specific stimulus (food, dyes, drugs, latex, cold, plants)

- **Differential diagnosis**: Angioedema (generalized swelling), erythema multiforme (spectrum of illness, the more severe forms of which have fever & mucous membrane lesions), contact dermatitis, mastocytosis, urticarial vasculitis

- **Acute urticaria**: Resolves <6 weeks. 80% acute urticaria resolve by 2 weeks.
- **Chronic urticaria**: 20% cases last >6 weeks. Of these, 50% resolve by 6 months.

- **Signs**: Pruritic, blanching, erythematous wheal surrounding pale/clear center.

- **Labs**: C-1 esterase inhibitor level for angioedema. Otherwise, direct tests towards suspected underlying etiology (anti-nuclear antibody, thyroid studies, etc)

- **Treatment**: 1st line therapy is a histamine receptor antagonist (H_1 or H_2)

Sedating H_1 antagonist	Diphenhydramine	5 mg/kg/d q 6-8hrs po (max 300 mg/day)
	Hydroxyzine	2 mg/kg/d q 6-8 hrs po (max 100 mg/day)
Non-sedating H_1 antagonist	Cetirizine	2-5 yrs: 2.5-5 mg daily po ≥6 yrs: 5-10 mg daily po
	Loratadine	2-5yrs: 5 mg daily po ≥6 yrs: 10 mg daily po
H_2 antagonist	Cimetidine	20-40 mg/kg/d divided q6 hrs (Max 300 mg/dose & 1200 mg/day)

H_1: Histamine-1 receptor; H_2: Histamine-2 receptor; po: orally

- Consider corticosteroids (1-2 mg/kg/day prednisone po; max 40 mg/day) for recalcitrant urticaria. Avoid prolonged use. Taper if symptoms recur when steroids stopped.

- **Referral**: To allergist for idiopathic, severe, recurrent, vasculitic, or chronic urticaria.

PRIMARY IMMUNODEFICIENCY (PI)

Suspect immunodeficiency when a child has:

> ≥8 ear infections, ≥2 sinus infections or 2 pneumonias in one year
> Family history of primary immunodeficiency
> Failure of an infant to appropriately gain weight
> Recurrent, deep skin or organ abscesses
> Persistent candidal infection in mouth or elsewhere on skin, after age 1
> Two or more months on antibiotics with little effect, or need for intravenous antibiotics to clear infections that normally would not require them

adapted from the Jeffrey Modell Foundation website: http://www.jmfworld.org/

Primary Immune Deficiency	Clinical Presentation
Severe combined immunodeficiency (SCID)	Infants present with failure to thrive, chronic diarrhea, recurrent opportunistic infections
Humoral (B-cell) immune defects	Sinopulmonary infections with encapsulated bacteria (S. pneumoniae, H. influenzae)
Selective IgA deficiency	Often asymptomatic. May have recurrent sinopulmonary infections, allergic reaction to blood products, autoimmune disorders
Cellular (T-cell) immune defects: DiGeorge syndrome, X-linked Hyper-IgM, Wiskott-Aldrich, Ataxia-telangiectasia	Opportunistic infections (cytomegalovirus, Pneumocystis jiroveci, mycobacteria)
Neutrophil defect: Chronic granulomatous disease (CGD)	Bacterial & fungal infections of skin and organs, including deep abscesses, granulomas, osteomyelitis, pneumonia
Complement Defect	Sinopulmonary infections with encapsulated bacteria and recurrent Neisseria infections
Interferon-gamma/interleukin-12 pathway defect	Atypical mycobacterial (include Bacillus Calmette-Guérin) and Salmonella infections

Immunodeficiency evaluation

▶ Growth parameters, CBC with differential, quantitative immunoglobulins, human immunodeficiency virus (HIV) testing
▶ Consider specific antibody titers after vaccination (H. influenzae, S. pneumoniae, tetanus), CH50 assay (tests complement function), neutrophil oxidation burst, consultation with immunologist.

Treatment:

May include antibiotic prophylaxis (trimethoprim-sulfamethoxazole for Pneumocystis), intravenous immunoglobulin* (humoral defects, hyper IgM, Wiskott-Aldrich), thymic transplantation (DiGeorge), bone marrow or stem cell transplantation (SCID), and/or interferon-gamma (CGD).

Fatal systemic infections can occur in patients with T cell defects who receive live vaccines such as Bacille Calmette-Guérin (BCG), oral polio vaccine (OPV), or measles/mumps/rubella vaccine (MMR).

*No live attenuated vaccines for at least 3 months after intravenous immunoglobulin (IVIG) due to poor vaccine response.

ALLERGIC RHINITIS

Classification of Allergic Rhinitis:

- *Mild:* No impairment in daily activities, school, sports, or sleep.
- *Moderate-severe:* Impairment in daily activities, school, sports, or sleep.
- *Intermittent:* Symptoms < 4days/ week or < 4 weeks duration.
- *Persistent:* Symptoms > 4 days/ week or > 4 weeks duration.

Medications used in the treatment of allergic rhinitis (based on age of patient)

Oral Antihistamines		
Diphenhydramine (*Benadryl*)	2-5 yrs old: 6.25 mg PO Q 4 hr 6-12 yrs old: 12.5 mg PO Q 4 hr > 12 yrs old: 12.5-25 mg q4 hr prn	•syrup: 12.5 mg/ 5 mL •chewable 12.5 mg •tablets 25 mg, 50 mg
Loratadine (*Claritin*)	2-5 yrs old: 5 mg PO daily > 6 yrs old: 10 mg PO daily	•syrup: 5mg/ 5 mL •tabs: 10 mg
Cetirizine (*Zyrtec*)	6-23 mo old: 2.5 mg PO daily 2-5 yrs old: 5 mg PO daily > 6 yrs old: 10 mg PO daily	•syrup: 5 mg/ 5 mL •tabs: 5, 10 mg •chewable: 5, 10 mg
Desloratadine (*Clarinex*)	6-11 mo old: 1 mg PO daily 1-5 yrs old: 1.25 mg PO daily 6-11 yrs old: 2.5 mg PO daily > 11yrs old: 5 mg PO daily	•syrup: 0.5 mg/ mL •tablets: 5 mg •RediTabs 2.5, 5 mg

Nasal Steroids*	
Budesonide (*Rhinocort-Aqua*)	•≥6 yrs old: 1-2 sprays each nostril daily
Fluticasone (*Flonase*)	•> 4 yrs old: 1-2 spray each nostril daily
Mometasone (*Nasonex*)	•2-11 yrs old: 1 spray each nostril daily •> 12 yrs old: 2 sprays each nostril daily
Triamcinolone (*Nasacort*)	•6-12 yrs old: 1-2 sprays/ nostril daily •>12 yrs old: 2 sprays/ nostril daily-BID

Leukotriene Inhibitors		
Montelukast (*Singulair*)	•6-23 mos old: 4 mg granules •2-5 yrs old: 4 mg PO •6-14 yrs old: 5 mg PO •> 14 yrs old: 10 mg PO	•granules: 4 mg packet •chewable: 4 mg, 5 mg •tablet: 10 mg (*All single daily dose*)

Intranasal Antihistamine		
Azelastine (*Astelin*)	•>5 yrs old: 1 puff/ nostril bid •>12 yrs old: 1-2 puff/nostril bid	•Seasonal allergic rhinitis •May cause sedation.

* One study showed ↓ linear growth in kids on nasal steroids (beclomethasone); another showed no effect in kids on budesonide, mometasone, or fluticasone.

IMMUNOTHERAPY: Consider if > 5 yrs old for systemic Hymenoptera reactions, pollens, dust mites, animal dander, cockroaches, fungi in severe cases; NOT used for eczema, urticaria, food or drug allergies.

Am J Med 10/06; 119(10): 820-3, *Immunol Allergy Clin North Am*, 2005; 25(2): 283-299.

FOOD ALLERGIES

PREVENTION: For high-risk infants (positive family history) consider:
▶ Avoiding peanuts while pregnant
▶ No dairy until 12 months (consider fully or partially hydrolyzed formula if not breastfed, see pp. 147-148); breastfeeding moms should consider cutting cow's milk, eggs, nuts (peanuts, almonds, walnuts) and fish out of diet.
▶ No eggs until 2 years old
▶ No nuts, fish/ seafood until 3 years old

RAST [radioallergosorbent test (blood test)] vs SKIN PRICK (Skin testing):
▶ *Skin prick* is gold standard for IgE-mediated disorders; less reliable in younger kids. Better negative predictive value (if negative test, more likely to not have allergy) than positive predictive value (if positive test, not absolute that there is an allergy).
▶ *RAST* can have specificity > 90% to certain foods (eggs, milk peanut, fish, soybean, wheat) with overall sensitivity 40-60 %. Sensitivity for fish is lower at 25%. Very high positive predictive value (if positive result, likely has allergy). If undetectable or very low specific IgE (<0.35 KIU/L), child unlikely to have allergy to specific food; but, some kids will have food allergy with negative test. Very high IgE are likely to be true allergens. Intermediate values may have unclear relevance.
▶ Total IgE: If ↑, may see more false positives to specific foods; if ↓ may see more false negatives for specific foods.

Allergen cross-reactivity:

Allergic to:	May also be allergic to:	Risk
Any legume	Another type of legume	5-10%
Any tree nut	Another type of tree nut	40%
Any fish	Another type of fish	50%
Any shellfish	Another type of shellfish	50-75%
Eggs	Chicken	5%
Cow's milk	Beef	10%
Cow's milk	Goat's milk	>90%
Pollen	Fruits/ vegetables	50%
Melon	Other fruits	90%
Latex	Fruit	35%
Fruit	Latex	10%

Adopted from Food Allergy in Children; Scurlock et al; Immunology and Allergy Clinics of North America May 2005

Cross reactivity of pollens- fruits in oral allergy syndrome

If allergic to:	May also be allergic to:
Ragweed	Melons/ bananas
Birch tree	Apple, carrots, kiwi
Mugwort	Celery

FOOD ALLERGY CONTINUED

TREATMENT:

▶ Eliminate allergen from diet (mother's diet if breastfed). For cow's milk allergy must also avoid artificial butter flavor, casein, pudding, ghee, hydrolysate, lactalbumin, nougat, whey & possibly brown sugar, caramel, chocolate, high protein flour, margarine.

▶ Soy formula can be considered after 6 months of age in IgE mediated allergy to cow's milk (less crossover than in non-IgE mediated disorders).

▶ Most non- IgE mediated disorders improve in 2-12 weeks after diet started.

▶ Oral challenges should be done in consultation with allergist.

▶ Use antihistamines for IgE mediated responses (urticaria, pruritus, anaphylaxis)

▶ Education and portable injectable epinephrine kit (Epi Pen) for kids who have possibility of anaphylaxis (even if no anaphylaxis on first episode, could on subsequent episodes). See Anaphylaxis management pp. 17

▶ Vaccines/ immunotherapy may be available in the future.

PROGNOSIS:

▶ If onset <3 years of age, more likely to outgrow within 2-3 years (milk, egg, soy, wheat).

▶ Sensitivity to allergen generally decreases with time, except for allergies to nuts & seafood. (20% will outgrow peanut allergy, but 8% will recur.)

▶ ↓IgE does not necessarily predict ↓allergic manifestations.

▶ *Risk factors for anaphylaxis*: Prior anaphylactic reaction; history of asthma; on angiotensin converting enzyme (ACE) inhibitor or beta-blocker; allergy to peanut, nuts, shellfish, fish.

RESOURCES:

www.wholesomebabyfood.com/allergy.htm, www.foodallergy.org, www.lpch.org/DiseaseHealthInfo/HealthLibrary/allergy/sitemap.html

REFERENCES:
American Academy of Pediatrics: Policy statement Hypoallergenic Infant Formulas, Pediatrics Vol. 106 No. 2 August 2000, pp. 346-349
Journal of Allergy and Clinical Immunology, Volume 116, Number 1, July 2005.
Immunology and Allergy Clinics of North America, Volume 25 (2), May 2005.

MANIFESTATIONS OF FOOD ALLERGY

Syndrome	Age	Symptoms	Foods	Risk factors	Other
Oral allergy syndrome	8-15 yrs	Itching mouth, tongue, palate immediately after eating food.	Raw melon, carrots, celery, potatoes, apples, bananas (often OK if cooked)	Allergic rhinitis (ragweed/ birch pollen)	Oral symptoms may precede allergic rhinitis symptoms.
Immediate GI hypersensitivity	Infant to child	Nausea, vomiting, abdominal pain within 2 hrs of food. Diarrhea later.	Milk, egg, peanut, soy, cereal, fish	Atopic dermatitis, asthma, allergic rhinitis	80% resolve (except fish & peanut) after eliminating dietary protein.
Skin symptoms	Infant/ child	Acute urticaria, angioedema, eczema	Milk, egg, fish, wheat, peanut, soy, tree nut	Up to 30% of kids with eczema have food allergy; may not improve by eliminating food.
Allergic eosinophilic gastro-enterocolitis	Infant to teens	Abdominal pain, anorexia, failure to thrive, gastro-intestinal bleeding, reflux, protein losing enteropathy	Milk, egg, fish, soy, cereals	Atopic dermatitis ↑IgE Eosinophilia (50%)	Skin test 50% specific; eosinophils on biopsy; 50% respond to food elimination/ hydrolyzed formula; usually persists.
Dietary protein enterocolitis	< 1 year	Bloody diarrhea, vomiting, anemia, failure to thrive	Milk, soy, poultry, fish, egg in older kids. (25% with intolerance to cow's milk also intolerant to soy)	Fecal leukocytes; normal IgE	Treat with elimination diet (breastfed) or hydrolyzed formula; 80% respond within 3-10 days. 20% require amino acid formula. 50% "outgrow" by 18 mos, 90% by 30 mos. Soy allergy may last longer.
Respiratory/ ocular symptoms	Infant/ child	Ocular pruritus, tearing, rhinorrhea, sneezing, cough, voice changes & wheeze	Eggs, milk, peanuts, tree nuts	Eczema, allergic rhinitis, asthma	IgE mediated

DEVELOPMENT			
Age	**Milestones/ behavior**	**Reflexes**	**Exam**
NEWBORN	Respond light/sound Flexion & adduction of extremities Fisted hand	Moro Grasp Galant Suck Root Stepping Deep tendon reflexes	Arm/leg recoil: full recoil normal Scarf sign: elbow stops at midline Heel to ear: not all the way to ear Popliteal angle: around 90° Ventral suspension: slumps Head lag: not fully flexed back Prone position: can turn head Note head circumference, shape, & sutures. Clonus may be normal in first weeks. Sustained is abnormal.
2-4 MONTHS	Social smile, laughs, squeals. tracks 180 degrees, bats objects, hands no longer fisted, holds object placed in hands. Hands to midline.	+Moro +ATNR *GONE:* Rooting Galant Stepping	Minimal head lag. Holds head upright when sitting. Head 45-90° off table if prone. Ventral suspension: Straight plane. Begins to bear weight on legs. Prone: Weight on forearms.
4-6 MONTHS	Smiles, jabbers Palmar grasp/ raking Sits with help Objects to mouth Transfers objects Rolls over (front to back usually first)	+/- Foot grasp *GONE:* Moro, Hand grasp	No head lag. Foot can reach mouth. Traction: Actively tries to sit. Prone: Chest off table, on hands. Bears weight on legs well (5 mo). Turns to voice (name). Imitates speech sounds.
6-9 MONTHS	Sits without support Pull to stand Stand holding on Mama/ dada Upset if left alone	Parachute Lateral Propping *GONE:* ATNR	Peek-a-boo Immature pincer grasp
9-12 MONTHS	Stranger anxiety Mama, dada specific Feeds self, pincer Wave bye-bye Crawls, creeps, walks	*GONE:* Plantar grasp	Toes up or downgoing Fine pincer grasp Gives kisses Protests when something taken away.

<u>**Primitive reflexes:**</u> (Persistence can be sign of upper motor neuron disease)
Moro: When drop head slightly (supported), both arms go out then in.
Gallant: Hold baby prone, stroke of back; tail end moves toward side stroked.
ATNR: When arm extended, head turns in same direction and opposite arm flexes.
Parachute: Hold baby prone and both arms will extend toward floor to support.

DEVELOPMENT CONTINUED

Developmental Milestones 1-5 years (See language development pp. 26)

Age	Social Milestones	Motor	Language
12-15 months	Imitate housework Uses utensils	Walking, stoops, scribbles	"Mama" "dada", + 3 words
15-18 months	Remove clothes Indicates wants ± Tantrums	Runs, kicks ball Walk backwards +/- handedness*	10 words, points to pictures/ body parts; greets with "Hi".
18-24 months	Wash hands	Throws ball, jump	½ understandable; 2 word phrases
2-3 years	Names a friend, puts on shirt	Draw line, balance 1 foot for 1 second	1 color, names 4 pictures
3-4 years	Brush teeth/ dresses alone	Copy circle, balance 2 seconds (1 foot)	Speech 100% understandable
4-5 years	Board games	Copy "+" sign; hops	Opposites

*Handedness does not develop until after 1 year; early lateralization may be sign of impaired control of the non-dominant hand.

DEVELOPMENTAL SCREENING: Ages and Stages Questionnaires®; Denver II Developmental Screening Test®; Parents Evaluation of Developmental Status (PEDS)

CAUSES OF DEVELOPMENTAL DELAY: Genetic disorders, prematurity/ birth complication, neurologic abnormality, idiopathic (see also topic on mental retardation pg. 25). If loss of skills present (regression), consider neurodegenerative disorders and inborn errors of metabolism.

WORKUP: Full physical and neurologic examination. Further workup as indicated by history and exam (highly variable). Consider consultation with neurologist, developmental specialist, physical/ occupational therapist as indicated.

RESOURCES: www.pathwaysawareness.org (checklist of normal development and red flags)

LANGUAGE DEVELOPMENT AND DELAY

▶ Receptive language (what child understands) develops before expressive language (what child can say).
▶ Language development is predictive of cognitive function. > 40% of kids with language delays will have learning problems.
▶ Hearing is critical to language development. Routine screening is recommended as history may miss 50% of kids with ↓ hearing.
▶ Language screening: Denver II, Early Language Milestones Scale. Parent self-screening tool: nidcd.nih.gov/health/voice/speechandlanguage.asp#mychild

DEVELOPMENT CONTINUED

NORMAL LANGUAGE DEVELOPMENT

Age	Questions to ask parents/ evaluate
0-5 months	React/ turns toward loud sounds. Responds when spoken to. Jabbers.
6-11 months	Imitates sounds, babbles, understand "NO", responds to name
12-17 months	Book/ story for ~ 2 minutes, points to objects, follow simple command with gestures. Mama/ dada specific by 15 months. > 5 words by 18 months, shows things to people.
18-23 months	10 words (+/- clear), follows simple directions without gestures, pronounces n, m, p, h and vowels, points to body parts, understands verbs like "eat", makes animal sounds, beginning to combine words
2 years old	~ 40-50 words, 2 words phrases, 50% intelligible
2-3 years	Pronouns (by 30 months), spatial relations ("in"), adjectives ("big"), plurals, and past tense. Speech ~75% understandable, >200 word vocabulary, 4-5 word sentences by 36 months.
3-4 years	Uses most speech sounds (may still have trouble with l, r, s, sh, ch, y, v, z, th until 6-7 years). Speech 100% understandable by 4. Answers simple questions. Knows colors and use of objects.
4-5 years	Understands > 1000 words, defines words, describes how to do things, rhyming.

Differential diagnosis of language delay: Developmental language disorder
  (improve with therapy), constitutional language delay ("late talker"), hearing loss,
  global developmental delay, pervasive developmental disorders/ autistic spectrum
  disorders, psychosocial deprivation or chronic illness. If regression of language
  skills consider Landau-Kleffner syndrome (abnormal electroencephalogram).
Factors that do not account for language delay: Older sibling; bilingual household
  (slight delay until 2-3 years old); boys may be *slightly* behind girls.

STUTTERING:

Risk Factors: Family history (60%), other developmental/ language problems, high
  stress/ fast paced lifestyle, male gender (3♂:1♀)
Prognosis: Better if stuttering develops before age 3 years, lasts < 6 months, ♀.
Indications for referral to speech/ language pathologist: Frequent stuttering (>
  10% of total language or > 3 per 100 syllables); long repetitions of sounds,
  syllables, and short words; frequent prolongations of sounds; consistent
  stuttering; persistent (duration >3-6 months); child appears stressed or has
  avoidant behaviors; parental or child concern
Resources: National Stuttering Association (www.westutter.org), American
  Speech-Language-Hearing Association (ASHA) (www.asha.org).

References: above websites, Dixon & Stein: Encounters with Children third edition 301-319; Weir Canadian Medical Association Journal Developmental disfluency: early intervention is key Volume 170, Number 12, June 8, 2004

SLEEP ISSUES IN CHILDHOOD: *Infants*

Average sleep times for children

Age	Nighttime Sleep	Daytime sleep
1 month	8-9 hours (1-4 hour naps)	7-8 hours (many naps)
3 months	6-10 hours	5-9 hours
6 months	10-12 hours	3-5 hours
12 months	11 hours	2-3 hours (2 naps)
2 years	11 hours	2 hours (1 nap)
3 years	11 hours	1-2 hours (1 nap)
4 years	11-12 hours	0
5-10 years	10-11 hours	0
10-16 years	8.5-10 hours	0

* adapted from University of Michigan Health System website: http://www.med.umich.edu/1libr/yourchild/sleep

▶ Infant sleep cycles are 50-60 minutes long; baby may wake with each cycle.
▶ < 4-6 months old, most babies will need $\geq$ 1 night feed, especially if breastfed.
▶ After 6 months, usually do not need to be fed and night-waking may be more behavioral. Baby needs to learn to put himself back to sleep without parents' help.
▶ There may be ↑in night waking with new developmental milestones (ie. walking).

Techniques for helping children sleep through the night:
▶ Keep regular daytime routine/ regular bedtime & night routine (bath, book, song).
▶ Avoid sleep onset associations (rocking/ nursing). May use to make child drowsy, but put in crib awake. Consider swaddling, pacifier, favorite blanket or stuffed animal.
▶ Curtains open/ time outside in daytime & dim lights, quiet at night.
▶ Ferber Method: involves allowing baby to "cry it out" at increasing intervals. Not generally recommended before 12-18 months of age. Short periods of crying with in-crib reassurance by parents may be effective after 6-9 months.
▶ Supplementing with formula or starting solids early do not necessarily make baby sleep longer.

Resources for parents regarding sleep issues:
▶ *The No-Cry Sleep Solution: Gentle Ways to Help Your Baby Sleep Through the Night*, by Elizabeth Pantley.
▶ *Solve your Child's Sleep Problems*, by Richard Ferber.
▶ *The Happiest Baby on the Block: The New Way to Calm Crying and Help Your Baby Sleep Longer*, by Harvey Karp.
▶ *Sleeping Through the Night*, by Jodi Mindell

References: *Child Care Health Dev* 1991 Sep-Oct;17(5):295-302; J Sleep Res. 2004 Dec;13(4):345-52.

SLEEP ISSUES IN CHILDHOOD: *older kids and adolescents*

Signs that older child needs more sleep:
Difficulty waking up in the morning
Difficulty falling asleep at night (requires more than 15-30 minutes)
Naps in daytime, or falls asleep in car or at school (10% of kids fall asleep @ school!)
Child may be hyperactive, irritable, moody, or have difficulty paying attention.

Sleep tips for children:
Keep a regular day and night sleep schedule, and have a bedtime routine
No TV, computer, or stimulating toys in bedroom
Avoid caffeinated drinks and snacks, especially at night
Make the child's bedroom comfortable, inviting, quiet and dark

Sleep disorders in Children:

Risk Factors: Presence of another sleep disorder, obstructive sleep apnea
   syndrome, nocturnal enuresis, family history, sleep deprivation, sedative
   medications, stress or illness.

NIGHT TERRORS, NIGHTMARES, SLEEP WALKING *(Somnambulism)*

Disorder	Age	Timing	Recall	Awake or asleep?
Night Terrors	3-12 yrs old	Early in sleep	No recollection	Can not comfort; child is asleep
Nightmares	Any age	Later in sleep	Recalls plot	Can comfort; child is awake
Sleep Walker	Any age	Deep sleep	No recollection	Asleep, but it is OK to wake child

Resources for parents:
1. National Sleep Foundation website: www.sleepfoundation.org
2. *Take Charge of Your Child's Sleep: The All-in-One Resource for Solving Sleep
   Problems in Kids and Teens*, by Judy Owens and Jodi Mindell.

DOWN SYNDROME

Incidence: Overall 1/600-700 births; ↑ risk with ↑ maternal age (1/385 at age 35)
Genetics: 95% trisomy 21. 3% are unbalanced translocation (25% familial); 1-2% mosaics (1 cell line normal, 1 cell line trisomy 21)

PHYSICAL FEATURES:

•One palmar crease •Brachycephalic head •Brushfield's spots •Protruding tongue	•Upslanting palpebral fissures •Wide space between 1st and 2nd toes •Short 5th finger, clinodactyly	•Hypotonia •↑ skin at back of neck •Epicanthal folds

ASSOCIATED CONDITIONS

•Mental retardation •Heart defects (50%) •Hearing loss (75%) •Celiac disease •Atlantoaxial instability	•Otitis media (50-70%) •Duodenal atresia •Thyroid disease (15%) •Eye disease (60%) •Hirschsprung's (1%)	•OSAS (50-75%) •Seizure disorder (5%) •Leukemia (1%) •Psychiatric conditions •Polycythemia (newborn)

OSAS= Obstructive Sleep Apnea Syndrome

CLINICAL CARE

Newborn	Evaluate for feeding problems, constipation, vomiting; hearing & newborn screen; screen for strabismus/ cataracts/ nystagmus; evaluate heart murmurs with echo; CBC; karyotype to confirm; Refer for support groups (National Down's Syndrome Society 800-221-4602; www.ndss.org) and special services.
1 month- 1 year	Thyroid function at 6-12 months old then annually. Ophthalmology by 6 months; Otolaryngology (ENT) referral if poor ear exam/ suspect anomaly/ failed hearing; behavioral audiometry by 1 year; plot growth on Down's syndrome growth chart (growthcharts.com); appropriate early intervention services; cardiology follow up as needed.
1-5 years	Audiometry every 6 months if stenotic ear canals; ENT as indicated; vision check yearly; cervical spine films (lateral flexion/ extension) once; thyroid screening annually; OSAS screening; school placement, behavior issues, special services.
5-13 years	Audio, ophthalmology, thyroid yearly. Consider celiac screening. Sexuality issues, gynecologic issues, social/ self help skills.
13-21 years	Annual audio, ophthalmology, thyroid function. CBC to screen for leukemia. Discuss & transition to adult medical care.

CBC= Complete Blood Count; ENT= otolaryngology; OSAS= Obstructive Sleep Apnea Syndrome;
PROGNOSIS: 15% die in first year; 50% live > 50 years.
Reference: AAP Policy: Health Supervision of Children with Down Syndrome (www.aap.org).

MENTAL RETARDATION (MR)

Definition: IQ (Intelligence quotient) < 70 AND deficits in functional & adaptive life skills.

Classification	IQ
Mild MR	55-70
Moderate MR	40-54
Severe MR	25-39
Profound MR	<25

Incidence: 1.6 - 3% of the population; 20% of people with MR have some degree of cerebral palsy. ↑risk psychiatric and seizure disorders in people with MR.

Presentation: Usually global developmental delay or isolated speech delay.

Etiology:
▶ Usually idiopathic
▶ Hundreds of genetic syndromes can have associated MR: Down syndrome, Fragile X, 5p- (cri-du-chat syndrome), 4p- (Wolf-Hirschhorn), Prader-Willi, Angelman, Smith-Magenis, DiGeorge and velocardiofacial syndrome, Williams syndrome, tuberous sclerosis, Smith-Lemli-Opitz, Rett syndrome, sex chromosome aneuploidy.
▶ Prenatal teratogen exposure (alcohol, drugs, anticonvulsants), lead, mercury, other heavy metal exposure, congenital hypothyroidism, metabolic disorders (especially if regression of milestones), structural brain disorders (microcephaly, hydrancephaly, agenesis of corpus callosum), hypoxic insult at birth, congenital infections, traumatic brain injury, prematurity (intraventricular hemorrhage), neurodegenerative disorders

Diagnosis: Thorough history, physical and neurologic exam.
▶ Psychological testing: Bayley Scales of Infant Development, Stanford Binet Intelligence Scale, Wechsler Intelligence Scale for Children (WISC) or Wechsler Preschool and Primary Scale of Intelligence (WPPSI)
▶ Labs and imaging may include (if indicated) karyotype, fluorescence in situ hybridization (FISH) probe for specific syndrome suspected, Fragile X probe (if + family history, physical findings). Metabolic screening if poor growth, vomiting, regression (urine organic acids, serum amino acids, urine mucopolysaccharides/ oligosaccharides); TSH/ Free T4; MRI or CT of the brain if developmental delay AND neurologic abnormality, macro/ microcephaly, or neurocutaneous findings.

Treatment: In most cases, educating family and optimizing educational and social resources is the mainstay of intervention.

Resources for parents: The Arc (www.thearc.org), Exceptional Parent Magazine (www.eparent.com)

References: Am Family Physician 2000; 61:1059-67,1070. Harum, Karen Dec 6, 2004 Mental Retardation

ATTENTION DEFICIT HYPERACTIVITY DISORDER (ADHD)

INCIDENCE: 6-9% of school aged kids. Can present with complaints of inattention/ hyperactivity/ impulsivity but parents may be concerned with school failure/ underachievement, low self esteem, problems with peers, oppositional behavior.

DIAGNOSIS: Must meet DSM criteria both at home and at school (or other non-home environment), with onset before 7 years of age. Behaviors must cause functional impairment (underachievement in school, difficulty with peers, problems with self esteem).

DSM-IV CRITERIA FOR ADHD- PREDOMINANTLY INATTENTIVE TYPE:
$\geq$6 of the following, for >6 months, developmentally inappropriate, and causing functional impairment.
1) Does not pay attention to details, or makes careless mistakes
2) Difficulty sustaining attention in tasks/ play
3) Does not seem to listen
4) Does not follow through or finish work
5) Avoids tasks that require sustained attention
6) Loses things
7) Easily distracted
8) Forgetful

DSM-IV CRITERIA FOR ADHD-PREDOMINANTLY HYPERACTIVE-IMPULSIVE TYPE: ($\geq$6 of the following for > 6 months duration)
HYPERACTIVITY:
1) Fidgets/ squirms
2) Leaves seat frequently when being seated is expected
3) Runs or climbs excessively when inappropriate
4) Difficulty playing/ engaging in leisure activities quietly
5) "On the go" or as if "driven by a motor"
6) Talks excessively

IMPULSIVITY:
1) Blurts out answers
2) Difficulty waiting for his/her turn
3) Frequently interrupts

DSM CRITERIA FOR COMBINED TYPE:
Child meets criteria for both inattentive and hyperactive/impulsive type.

▶ Information can be obtained by interview and questionnaires or narrative from teacher, parent or other caregiver. If possible, after obtaining parental consent, contact teacher directly. Questionnaires and other info at: www.nichq.org/NICHQ/Topics/ChronicConditions/ADHD/Tools/

ADHD CONTINUED

▶ *Comorbidities:* Oppositional defiant disorder (ODD) (30%), conduct disorder (CD) (25%), anxiety (20%), depression (20%), learning disabilities (15%), sleep disturbances (before medications started), substance use/ smoking.

DIFFERENTIAL DIAGNOSIS

• Social/ situational stress	• Absence seizures
• Adjustment reaction	• Hearing/ vision deficits
• Specific learning disability (requires psychoeducational testing for diagnosis)	• Sleep disturbance (includes OSAS)
	• Allergic rhinitis/ other medical problems
• Oppositional defiant disorder	• Hypo/ hyperthyroidism
• Anxiety disorders	• Medication side effects (steroids, β-agonists); substance use/ abuse
• Depression	• Fragile X syndrome
• Bipolar disorder (suspect if extreme, unprovoked tantrums/ outbursts, family history, decreased need for sleep, agitation)	• Fetal alcohol spectrum disorders, intrauterine drug exposure

OSAS: Obstructive Sleep Apnea Syndrome

WORKUP:

▶ Complete vital signs, hearing and vision screen, neurologic and physical exam should be done on all patients to evaluate for any underlying medical problem and as a baseline.

▶ Labs or other studies generally not indicated unless specific medical condition suspected.

TREATMENT: Identify specific goals and treatment outcome for each patient.

▶ School should be involved with 504 plan or Individual Education Plan (IEP). These may include psychoeducational testing, psychological evaluation, classroom accommodations, daily progress notes, extended testing times, etc.

▶ Medication +/- behavioral therapy is most effective. 80% of ADHD kids respond to one of the stimulant medications, though it may not be the first one tried.

▶ Start at low dose and increase every 4-7 days until desired effect attained and no/ minimal side effects. May start with short acting medication and change to long acting once dose is determined; or, may start with long acting stimulant (especially in older kids).

▶ Contraindications to medications include known allergy to the medication, or use of monoamine oxidase inhibitors. Use with caution in kids with cardiovascular disease, seizure disorder, tics, or marked anxiety.

▶ Stimulant side effects: ↓appetite, insomnia, stomach upset/ headache (↓ after 1-2 weeks). Monitor weekly when initiating/ titrating medication; check height, weight, heart rate and blood pressure every 3-6 months once at a stable dose.

ADHD CONTINUED

MEDICATIONS USED IN THE TREATMENT OF ADHD: FIRST LINE AGENTS

DRUG (duration)	DOSE RANGE	DOSAGE FORMS	OTHER
Methylphenidate (MPH) Options			
Ritalin (3-4 hrs)	Start with 5 mg in morning. MAX 60 mg/day.	5 mg, 10 mg, 20 mg. Scored tablets.	Add noon dose and ↑5 mg/ week to effect.
Methylin (3-4 hrs)	Start:5 mg in a.m. Max 60 mg/day.	Solution: 5 mg/5 ml or 5 mg/10 mL Chewable tabs: 2.5, 5, 10 mg	
Long Acting Methylphenidate Options			
Ritalin LA (6-8 hrs) Ritalin SR (4-8 hrs)	Start with 20 mg daily; MAX 60 mg/day	Ritalin LA: 20 mg,30 mg, 40 mg capsules; Ritalin SR: 20 mg	Can sprinkle; may need afternoon dose
Metadate ER/CD (4-8 hrs)	Start with 10mg daily; MAX 60 mg/day.	ER: 10mg, 20 mg tabs; CD: 10, 20, 30, 40, 50 60 mg tabs.	May need to add afternoon dose.
Methylin ER (8 hrs)	Start with 10 mg single daily dose.	10 mg, 20 mg tabs; MAX 60mg/day	
Concerta (8-12 hrs)	Start with 18mg, MAX 72 mg.	18 mg, 27 mg, 36 mg, 54 mg	Do not open capsule.
Dexmethylphenidate hydrochloride			
Focalin (3-4 hrs)	Start with 2.5 mg in morning; MAX 20 mg/day.	2.5 mg, 5 mg, 10 mg tablets. (2x potency of MPH)	Add noon dose and ↑2.5-5 mg/ week to effect.
Focalin XR (8-12 hrs)	Start with 5mg single daily dose; MAX 20 mg.	5 mg (blue), 10 mg (yellow), 20 mg (white) capsules.	Can open capsule & sprinkle.
Dextroamphetamine + amphetamine			
Adderall (4-6 hrs)	Start with 5 mg 1- 2x/ day. Max 30mg/day	5 mg, 7.5 mg, 10 mg, 12.5 mg, 15 mg, 20mg, 30 mg tabs	↑ by 5 mg/ week to desired effect.
Adderall XR (8-12 hrs)	Start with 5 mg, MAX 30mg/day	5, 10, 15, 20, 25, 30 mg capsules	Can sprinkle
Atomoxetine			
Strattera (24 hours)	Start with 0.5 mg/kg/day; MAX 1.4 mg/kg/day.1-2 doses per day.	Tablets: 10,18, 25, 40, 60, 80, 100 mg (max 80 for most adolescents)	Nausea, ↓appetite, *beware suicidal thoughts
Lisdexamfetamine			
Vyvanse	30 mg daily, MAX 70 mg daily	30, 50, 70 mg capsules	Studied in kids aged 6-12 yrs

ADHD CONTINUED

SECOND LINE AGENTS

DRUG	DOSE RANGE	DOSE FORMS	OTHER
Daytrana Patch* (3-12 hours)	Start with 10 mg, max 30 mg daily. Lower dose than oral equivalent.	10 mg, 15 mg, 20 mg, 30mg	Lasts 3 hours after patch removed; studied in kids aged 6-12 yrs.
Bupropion (4-8 hours)	Start with 37.5 mg daily; ↑ to BID	75 mg, 100 mg (MAX 150 mg/ dose)	Side effects: ↓ appetite, insomnia, irritable mood;
Bupropion sustained release (10+ hours)	Start with 100 mg daily	100 mg, 150 mg, 200 mg	may ↓ seizure threshold?

THIRD LINE AGENTS

Clonidine** (3-6 hours)	Start with 0.025-0.05 mg/day at night, ↑ weekly; MAX 0.3 mg/ day.	0.1, 0.2,0.3 mg tablets; give 1-4 doses/day.	Most effective for impulsive/ hyperactive; taper off to avoid rebound hypertension.
Guanfacine (6-12 hours)	Start with 0.5 mg/day	1,2,3mg tabs	Less side effects than clonidine

*Second line because ~25% have skin rash; could cause sensitization to oral methylphenidate. Use in kids who cannot swallow medication.

**Clonidine side effects: Sleepiness, hypotension, headache, dizziness, or nausea.

MEDICATION TROUBLESHOOTING & TREATING COEXISTING CONDITIONS

Tics	Can try to ↓dose or add/change to clonidine, guanfacine
Anxiety	*Strattera* (may be more effective in ADHD + anxiety than stimulants) or bupropion
Depression	Bupropion; stimulant + selective serotonin reuptake inhibitor; *Strattera*
Weight loss	↑calorie foods in AM & PM; nutrition shakes; decrease dose or Δ medication
Insomnia	No caffeine, no TV in room, routine before bed; use ↓duration stimulant, melatonin 1-1.5 mg before bed, clonidine before bed.
Med wears off/ rebound	Use long-acting stimulant; or, add short-acting stimulant in evening; or, try *Strattera* (0.5 mg/kg/day) + stimulant; or, split long-acting ½ dose in AM, ½ at noon.
Child 3-5 years	Parent training, structured preschool, behavioral therapy; if use med, consider low-dose methylphenidate & titrate up to effect.

References: AAP Policy statement on ADHD (www. aap.org); Consultant for Pediatricians 8/06 5:8

DEPRESSION

RISK FACTORS: family/ personal history of depression; social/academic stress; chronic illness; any coexisting disorder listed below.

DIAGNOSIS: May present with subtle problems at school/ with peers, somatic complaints, high-risk behavior. Thorough history, family history, and context of problems are key. Consult child psychologist/psychiatrist if beyond comfort level.

▶ *Differential diagnosis*: Dysthymic disorder, substance use, bereavement, adjustment reaction, underlying medical condition, post-traumatic stress disorder (PTSD); **MUST rule out Bipolar Disorder.**

> *Major Depressive Episode*: ≥ 2 weeks of depressed mood or loss of interest/pleasure plus 4 or more of: 1) appetite change, 2) sleep disturbance, 3) psychomotor agitation/retardation, 4) ↓ energy, 5) worthlessness/guilt, 6) ↓ concentration, 7) thoughts of death/ suicide. Must NOT be a mixed episode, bereavement or drug effect. Must cause significant impairment in functioning.

> *Dysthymic disorder*: Depressed mood most days for 1 yr plus ≥ 2 of: 1) appetite Δ, 2) sleep Δ, 3)↓ energy, 4)↓ self esteem, 5)↓ concentration, 6) ↓hope

COMORBIDITIES (majority have ≥ 1): Anxiety disorders, ADHD, oppositional defiant disorder, substance use/ abuse, eating disorders, learning disabilities.

TREATMENT:

▶ Treatment for Adolescents with Depression Study (TADS) showed 35% responded to placebo, 43% to cognitive behavioral therapy (CBT) alone, 60% responded to fluoxetine alone, and 71% responded to fluoxetine + CBT (↓ doses of fluoxetine were needed in this group)

▶ Trial of cognitive behavioral therapy alone may be considered if nonsevere.

▶ *Medications*: Carefully discuss risks/ benefits with patient/ family. Face to face contact weekly x 1-2 mo. Educate about emergency contacts (suicidehotlines.com)

▶ **www.parentsmedguide.org** (by APA and AACAP for physicians and parents)

> **Fluoxetine** is the only selective serotonin reuptake inhibitor (SSRI) approved for kids (> 8 years old). Start with 2.5-10 mg/day; May take 4 weeks to develop full effect; titrate slowly. Taper off. Available in 10 mg scored tabs; 10, 20, 40 mg pulvules; 20 mg/5 mL liquid; Caution if renal, hepatic, cardiac dysfunction, seizure disorder; Side effects: Headache, dizziness, sedation, sleep Δ, nausea.

▶ Black box warning on antidepressant medications issued by FDA 10/04. Suicidal thoughts in 4% on meds versus 2% on placebo. No completed suicides. No evidence that meds ↑ suicide, but studies suggest that treating depression overall decreases risk of suicide.

PROGNOSIS: 9/10 teens recover within 2 years; risk of relapse & adult depression. Suicide risk factors: Previous attempt, severe depression, clear plan for suicide.

Reference: Ferren, P, *Contemporary Peds* 23:2 2/2006; TADS *J Am Acad Child Adolesc Psychiatry* - 01-DEC-2006

TICS/ TOURETTE'S SYNDROME (TS)

<u>TIC</u>: Sudden, repetitive movement or verbalization; tends to ↑ with stress/ fatigue and ↓ with sleep and concentration. Tics are often temporarily suppressible.

<u>MOTOR TICS</u>: Simple: Eye blinking, head jerk; Complex: Slapping, tapping, punching, biting. Can be isolated or early manifestation of Tourette's Syndrome.

<u>VERBAL TICS</u>: Simple: Throat clearing, grunting, sniffing; Complex: Acute change in rate/ volume of speech, echolalia, talking to oneself, obscene speech (rare).

"Intentional repetitive behavior": Often difficult to tell the difference between complex tic and compulsion; much overlap between obsessive compulsive disorder (OCD) and Tourette's.

<u>TRANSIENT</u>: < 1 year; <u>CHRONIC</u>: > 1 year (< 3 consecutive months tic free)

<u>TOURETTE'S SYNDROME</u>: Both multiple motor tics and vocal tics; typical onset at 5-10 years old (simple motor tics →vocal tics later); tends to peak in adolescence but may improve later in life. Must have onset < 18 yrs for diagnosis; lasts > 1 yr.

<u>COMORBIDITIES</u>: Attention deficit hyperactivity disorder (ADHD; 50% with TS), OCD (25-40% with TS), trichotillomania, mood and anxiety disorders, ~70% with TS have some type of behavior problem and 30% with TS have learning problems.

<u>INHERITANCE</u>: ↑incidence in families with Tourette's syndrome, OCD.

<u>Pediatric autoimmune neuropsychiatric disorder associated with group A streptococci (PANDAS)</u>: Children who develop or have worsening of OCD or tic disorders after an infection with Group A Strep.

<u>RISK FACTORS</u>: Male, family history of Tourette's syndrome or OCD, perinatal complications, high prenatal exposure to coffee, nicotine or alcohol.

<u>TREATMENT</u>: *Mild*: Education, support, behavioral interventions (habit reversal: developing alternate behavior to perform when patient feels a tic coming on); *Severe*: In addition to above consider medications.

Medication	Dose	Side effects	Notes	Forms
Clonidine (alpha-adrenergic agonist)	0.1-0.3 mg / day divided 1-4 times/ day	Sedation, hypotension, dizziness	Not currently FDA approved for this purpose; wean when stopping medication.	Tabs or patch: 0.1, 0.2 0.3 mg
Guanfacine	0.5-3 mg/day divided 1-4 times/day	Sedation, constipation, hypotension	Do not use if renal/ cardiac condition, or bradycardia. Monitor blood pressure & pulse.	1 mg or 2 mg tablets
Antipsychotics (haloperidol, pimozide, risperidone, olanzapine)	Variable depending on agent	Sedation, weight gain, acute dystonic reactions	Generally considered second line because of higher incidence of side effects.	Variable

Resources: www.tsa-usa.org, www.tourettesyndrome.net
References: *Tourette's Syndrome*, Psychiatric Clinics of North America, 2006(29) Number 2

ENCOPRESIS

Encopresis with constipation (95%)	**Encopresis without constipation (5%)**
Functional (95%)	*Nonorganic* (99%): Potty training resistance, toilet phobia, stress
Organic (<5%): Anal fissure, trauma;	*Organic*: Inflammatory bowel disease, diarrhea, spinal cord tumor, fistula, trauma
Neurologic: Hirschsprung's, spinal cord disorder, pelvic mass	
Other: Hypothyroidism, ↑calcium, lead, drugs	

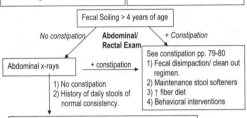

Fecal Soiling > 4 years of age

No constipation ← **Abdominal/ Rectal Exam** → *+ Constipation*

Abdominal x-rays

+ constipation

1) No constipation
2) History of daily stools of normal consistency.

See constipation pp. 79-80
1) Fecal disimpaction/ clean out regimen.
2) Maintenance stool softeners
3) ↑ fiber diet
4) Behavioral interventions

Workup based on exam findings (see differential above).
If nonorganic → counseling and /or behavioral interventions.

Behavioral Interventions (general): Ensure soft stools. Provide incentives/ rewards for appropriate use of toilet. When soils, help to change quickly. Do not scold. Schedule toilet sits (3-5 x/ day), especially after meals. Ensure safe/ non-ridiculed toileting environment (like might happen at school).
Potty Training Resistance: Give child all potty control; minimize use of diapers & Pull Ups®
Toilet Phobia: Parent modeling, scheduled toilet "sits", associate toilet time with fun and positive parent interaction. Start with short toilet sits with clothes on and gradual ↑ time on toilet and pants off.

POTTY TRAINING

POTTY TRAINING READINESS: (typically by 24-30 months of age)
► Sphincter control usually present by the time child walks.
► Can child walk to and sit on toilet, pull down pants, flush & stay dry for hours?
► Can child communicate that he/ she needs to go to the toilet?
► Is child curious about "poo poo" and "pee pee" or genitals?
► Does child have desire to please parents and follow directions?

American Family Physician 1999; 59 (8); 2171-2182; Stein, Dixon Encounters with Children 3rd edition

ENURESIS

PRIMARY NOCTURNAL ENURESIS

▶ Child > 5 years old wets bed ≥ 2x/ week & has never been consistently dry at night. 25% of 4 year olds, 10% of 8 year olds, 3% of 12 year olds wet bed.
▶ Risk: 15% if no family history; 44% if one parent affected; 77% if both parents.
▶ Rule out: Urinary tract infection (UTI), sleep apnea, neurologic/ spinal cord abnormality, and fecal impaction.
▶ Red flags: Daytime wetting/ urgency, abnormal exam, + urinalysis, history of UTI
▶ Interventions: Fluid restriction after dinner and/or scheduled night waking to urinate.
▶ *Bedwetting alarms* highest success (70%). If no ↓ at 3 months, try medications.
▶ *Desmopressin:* Nasal spray 100 mcg/mL (10 mcg/spray), 1-4 sprays before bed; 0.2 mg tablets; 0.2-0.6 mg po before bed. Approved ≥ 6 years old. 80% relapse.
▶ *Imipramine:* (> 6 years old) 1-2.5 mg/kg/day po at bedtime [max 50 mg (6-12 years) or 75 mg (>12 years)]. Treat for 4-6 months. Consider EKG prior to initiation; Caution if heart disease, seizure disorder. 50% relapse rate.

SECONDARY NOCTURNAL ENURESIS

▶ Recurrence of night wetting after > 6 months dry, often after stress or trauma.

DIURNAL ENURESIS/ VOIDING SYMPTOMS

▶ Occasional daytime "accidents" common; evaluate if frequent or persistent.
▶ *Differential diagnosis*: UTI, constipation/ impaction, spinal cord abnormalities/ neurogenic bladder, posterior urethral valves, anatomic anomalies, diabetes insipidus or mellitus, or others listed in chart below.
▶ *Thorough history and physical exam*: External genitalia, abdomen (for mass), rectal exam, lumbosacral spine (dimple, hair tuft) & neurologic exam.
▶ *Evaluation*: At a minimum, urinalysis (culture if indicated), renal ultrasound (RUS), and voiding cystourethrogram (VCUG) should be done. Thickened bladder wall, hydronephrosis, or significant post-void residual suggests obstruction. Refer to urology for urodynamic studies if indicated.

Syndrome	Symptoms	RUS	VCUG	Other
Infrequent voiding	Does not void for 8-12 hours	Normal	Normal	Frequent void program
Fecal Impaction	Wetting	Normal	Normal	Treat constipation
Giggle incontinence	Wets with laughing	May see ↑detrusor activity on urodynamics		↑voiding
Vaginal reflux	Dribble	Normal	Vaginal urine	Sit backwards on toilet to void
Daytime frequency	Urgency and frequency	Normal	Normal	Resolves over months

Walsh: Campbell's Urology, 8th ed., 2002 Saunders Section B: Non-Neurogenic Lower Urinary Tract Dysfunction; *Journal of the American Academy of Child and Adolescent Psychiatry* 43: 12, December 2004

AUTISTIC SPECTRUM DISORDERS (ASD)

EPIDEMIOLOGY:
▶ Most likely, genetic plus environmental factors contribute to development of ASD
▶ 75% concordance in monozygotic twins; 3% in dizygotic twins; 3-6% non-twin siblings
▶ Associated disorders include Fragile X syndrome, tuberous sclerosis (1- 4%), untreated phenylketonuria (PKU), and congenital rubella syndrome.
> <u>Fragile X</u>: Up to 10% of kids with ASD have Fragile X syndrome; in those families, 50% recurrence risk in future boys born to same parents.
> <u>Landau-Kleffner Syndrome</u>: Language regression between 3-6 years of age and abnormal EEG, but without other autistic features.

▶ Association with vaccines: Several large-scale studies in different countries do not show any link between measles-mumps-rubella (MMR) vaccine and autism.
▶ <u>Thimerosal</u> is unlikely to be a cause of autism, as several studies showed continued increase in autism diagnosis after it was removed from vaccines.
▶ Unclear role of associated gastrointestinal disorders, immune responses, and allergies.

FEATURES: (please refer to DSM-IV for specific diagnostic criteria)
▶ All ASD's exhibit impaired social interaction/ ability to relate, impaired language as used in social contexts, and restricted/ repetitive behavior patterns or interests.
▶ There is a spectrum of disorders, ranging from mild (Asperger syndrome) to severe (Autism, Childhood Disintegrative Disorder).
▶ May be associated with mental retardation, seizure disorder, macrocephaly.

The Autistic Spectrum Disorders

Disorder	Features
Autistic Disorder	Impaired social interaction, communication, & imaginative play and stereotyped behaviors with onset before 3 years. 75% have mental retardation.
Asperger Syndrome	Average to above-average intelligence and no speech delay (though still abnormalities in use of pragmatic speech). May have fine motor coordination problems.
Pervasive Developmental Disorder NOS	Impaired social/ communication skills, stereotyped behaviors/ interests, but late onset or criteria not met for diagnosis of autistic disorder.
Rett Syndrome	After period of normal development, mental and social regression and deceleration of head growth at 5-48 months; hand wringing. Almost all affected are female.
Childhood Disintegrative Disorder (CDD)	Normal development until 2-4 years, followed by loss of motor, language and social skills.

NOS= Not otherwise Specified

| AUTISTIC SPECTRUM DISORDERS CONTINUED |

SCREENING: Primary physicians should screen all patients at well visits.
▶ Screening instruments: The Modified Checklist for Autism in Toddlers (M-CHAT) at 12 month visit (available at www.firstsigns.org), the Social Communication Questionnaire (SCQ) (for children ≤4 years), The Autism Spectrum Screening Questionnaire (ASSQ), Childhood Asperger Syndrome Test (CAST).
▶ Red flags include language delay, no joint attention (2 kids paying attention to same object at same time), no pointing to indicate interest, no bringing things to parent to show them, poor eye contact, poor response to name.

DIAGNOSIS: Early diagnosis and intervention lead to improved outcomes. Clinical diagnosis best made by multidisciplinary team including psychologist, psychiatrist, neurologist, speech/ language pathologist, etc. Standardized instruments may be used including Autism Diagnostic Interview (ADI-R) and Autism Diagnostic Observation Schedule

OTHER STUDIES TO CONSIDER

▶ Audiology evaluation ▶ Lead level ▶ Phenylketonuria (PKU) screen ▶ Fragile X testing/ chromosomal analysis ▶ Neuropsychological testing (ie. IQ)	▶ CT, MRI, positron emission tomography scan, and EEG not routinely recommended, but may be indicated in certain situations.

TREATMENT:

▶ Behavioral interventions: Mainstay of treatment for ASD. Language, occupational, physical and social play therapies are integral parts of a comprehensive program. A predictable schedule, structured activities, regular reinforcement and parental involvement are keys to program success.

▶ Medications: Medications may help with specific undesirable behaviors. They should be used with caution as effects unpredictable in kids with ASD. Consider consultation with pediatric neurologist or psychiatrist.
   •*Hyperactivity*: Stimulant medications may be helpful in some kids[1], but ↑ risk of irritability, anxiety and other side effects. Atomoxetine may be useful in some kids[1]. Alpha$_2$ agonists may also be considered but no good large-scale studies[2].
   •*Obsessions, compulsions, adherence to routine, anxiety, mood disorders*: Some selective serotonin reuptake inhibitors have been used with some benefit, but may cause agitation, hyperactivity, and hypomania.[2]
   •*Aggression, irritability and self injurious behavior*: Risperidone is FDA approved for this purpose. Side effects include weight gain, and fatigue.

1. *J Am Acad Child Adolesc Psychiatry*, 2006; 45(10): 1196-205. 2. *J Clin Psychiatry*, 2005:66 Suppl 10

AUTISTIC SPECTRUM DISORDERS CONTINUED

Risperidone dosing for kids > 5 years old with ASD

Weight	Starting Dose	Titration Schedule	Most Effective Dose
< 20 kg	0.25 mg PO daily (1-2 doses/day)	After 4 days, increase to 0.5 mg daily; then q 2 weeks by 0.25 mg daily prn.	1 mg PO daily
20-45 kg	0.5 mg PO daily (1-2 doses/ day)	After 4 days, increase to 1 mg PO daily, then q 2 weeks by 0.5 mg daily prn.	2.5 mg PO daily
> 45 kg	0.5 mg PO daily (1-2 doses/ day)	After 4 days, increase to 1 mg PO daily, then q 2 weeks by 0.5 mg daily prn.	3 mg PO daily

▶ Diet: Some reports suggest that eliminating certain food (primarily gluten and casein) from one's diet may help autistic behaviors, but no large, well controlled studies have been done to date.

RESOURCES FOR PARENTS AND PROFESSIONALS

www.autism-society.org, www.autism-pdd.net, www.maapservices.org

FRAGILE X SYNDROME

▶ Most common inheritable form of mental retardation; 1:3600 males and 1:5000 females affected; 1:800 men and 1:300 women are carriers. 3-6% of autistic kids also have fragile X syndrome.
▶ Signs: Learning disabilities, mental retardation, pervasive developmental disorders/ autistic spectrum disorders. Physical stigmata: Long face, large ears, macroorchidism, loose ligaments, flat feet, mitral valve prolapse.
▶ Diagnosis: DNA analysis "FMR-1 gene test" [using both polymerase chain reaction (PCR) and southern blot]
▶ Treatment: Educational services; speech, physical, occupational therapy; sensory integration therapy, medications aimed at specific symptoms may be helpful.
▶ Resources: www.fragilex.org

ARRHYTHMIAS & ECG INTERPRETATION

Normal ECG Values

Age	P-R interval[a]	QRS interval[a]	QRS axis (mean)	QTc[b]
0-7 days	0.08-0.12	0.04-0.08	80-160 (125)	0.34-0.54
1-4 weeks	0.08-0.12	0.04-0.07	60-160 (110)	0.30-0.50
1-3 months	0.08-0.12	0.04-0.08	40-120 (80)	0.32-0.47
3-6 months	0.08-0.12	0.04-0.08	20-80 (65)	0.35-0.46
6-12 months	0.09-0.13	0.04-0.08	0-100 (65)	0.31-0.49
1-3 years	0.10-0.14	0.04-0.08	20-100 (55)	0.34-0.49
3-8 years	0.11-0.16	0.05-0.09	40-80 (60)	< 0.45
8-16 years	0.12-0.17	0.05-0.09	20-80 (65)	< 0.45

[a] seconds [b] QTc = QT interval / (square root of preceding RR interval); reported in seconds

ECG Diagnosis of Chamber Enlargement (Hypertrophy)

Right ventricular hypertrophy (RVH) • R in V1 > 20 mm (> 25 mm < 1 mo) • S in V6 > 6 mm (> 12 mm < 1 mo) • Upright T in V3R, V1 after 5 day • QR pattern in V3R, V1	**Biventricular hypertrophy** • RVH and (S in V1 or R in V6) exceeding mean for age • LVH and (R in V1 or S in V6) exceeding mean for age
Left ventricular hypertrophy (LVH) • R in V6 > 25 mm (> 21 mm < 1 yr) • S in V1 > 30 mm (> 20 mm < 1 yr) • R in V6 + S in V1 > 60 mm (use V5 if R in V5 > R in V6) • Abnormal R/S ratio • S in V1 > 2 X R in V5	**Right atrial hypertrophy** • Peak P value > 3 mm (< 6 months), > 2.5 mm (≥ 6 months) **Left atrial hypertrophy** • P in II > 0.09 seconds • P in V1 with late negative deflection > 0.04 seconds and > 1 mm deep

ECG Findings in Medical Disorders

Disorder	Typical ECG Findings (not necessarily most common)
Calcium	Hyper - short QT, AV block, ↓ HR, Hypo - long QT, ↑ HR
CNS bleed	Diffuse deep T inversion, prominent U, QT > 60% of normal
Digoxin effect	Downward curve of ST segment, flat/inverted T's, short QT
Hyperkalemia	Peaked T's, wide then flat P's, wide QRS and QT, sine wave
Hypokalemia	Flat T waves, U waves, ST depression
Thyroid	Hypo - ↓ HR, ↓ voltage, ST ↓, flat/↓ T waves; Hyper-↑ HR
Kawasaki disease	Prolonged P-R, nonspecific ST-T changes
Lyme disease	AV block, pericarditis, intraventricular conduction delays
Myocarditis	Diffuse nonspecific ST-T △, AV block, ventricular ectopy
Pericarditis	Diffuse ST elevation, PR segment depression, ↓ voltage

Reprinted with permission, Tarascon Pediatric Emergency Pocketbook
5th Edition, Tarascon Publishing, Lompoc, CA, 2007.

CARDIAC MURMURS

Consider pediatric cardiology consultation for: Abnormal ECG, abnormal size/shape of cardiac silhouette on chest x-ray, ≥III/VI systolic murmur, cyanosis, abnormal pulses or heart sounds, grunting & poor feeding in infant, diastolic murmur.

Classification based on intensity:

• *Grade I*: Barely audible	• *Grade V*: Audible with stethoscope barely on
• *Grade II*: Soft, easily audible	chest
• *Grade III*: Loud, no thrill	• *Grade VI*: Audible with stethoscope off chest
• *Grade IV*: Loud, +thrill	

Innocent murmurs	Description	Age at auscultation
Branch pulmonary stenosis	Systolic, upper left sternal border, I-II/VI intensity, transmits to axillae & back. If persists, consider pulmonic stenosis.	Infants, up to 3-6 mos
Still's murmur	Systolic, left lower-mid sternal border, II-III/VI, vibratory, low-frequency	3-6 yrs
Venous hum: (turbulence in jugular)	Continuous, I-III/VI, right or left supra/infraclavicular areas. Differentiate from patent ductus arteriosus (PDA)	3-6 yrs
Carotid bruit	Systolic, right supraclavicular and carotid, II-III/VI, occasional thrill	Any age
Pulmonary ejection murmur	Early-mid systolic ejection, I-III/VI, no radiation	8-14 yrs

Pathologic murmurs	Description	Location
Patent ductus arteriosus	Continuous, II-IV/VI, possible bounding pulses, louder with ↓pulmonary resistance	Left infraclavicular
Ventricular septal defect	Holosystolic, "blowing", II-V/VI, louder with ↓pulmonary resistance	Left lower sternal border
Atrial septal defect	Systolic, II-III/VI, widely split & fixed S2	Left upper sternal border
Pulmonic stenosis	Systolic ejection, II-V/VI, S2 widely split, ejection click	Left upper sternal border & back
Aortic stenosis	Systolic ejection, II-V/VI, ejection click	Right upper sternal border
Mitral valve prolapse	Systolic, II-III/VI	Mid-precordium→left axilla.

• **Absence of murmur** does not preclude serious heart anomalies.

• Neonates with ductal dependant lesions (transposition of the great arteries, pulmonary atresia, total anomalous pulmonary venous return) will present with cyanosis as ductus arteriosus closes.

• Congestive heart failure (from silent atrial septal defect, aberrant origin of coronary artery) as indicated by failure to thrive, sweating, tachypnea, may be presenting sign of structural heart lesion in older infants and children.

VENTRICULAR SEPTAL DEFECTS (VSD)

Most common congenital heart defect. Presentation depends on size of defect.
<u>Small VSD</u>: Asymptomatic, normal growth, watching and waiting is appropriate.
<u>Moderate-large VSD</u>: Often develop congestive heart failure (CHF) by 2-4 months
of age, resulting in tachypnea, poor feeding, excessive sweating, irritability.
Long-standing left→right shunt results in pulmonary hypertension (HTN).
Types of VSD: Membranous (60-70%), muscular (5-20%), inlet (~5%), outlet (~5%)

	Membranous	Muscular	Inlet defect	Outlet defect
Spontaneous closure	30-40%	35%	0%	0%

ATRIAL SEPTAL DEFECTS (ASD)

Often asymptomatic congenital defect with bidirectional flow across atrial septum.
<u>3 main types</u>: Secundum (50-70%), Primum (15-30%), Sinus venosus (10%).
Small % of ASD associated with partial anomalous pulmonary venous return.
<u>Exam</u>: Fixed split S2, possible diastolic murmur (↑blood across tricuspid valve),
pulmonic stenosis murmur, or lift from right ventricular enlargement.
<u>Diagnostic studies</u>: Chest X-ray may show enlarged right heart silhouette;
electrocardiogram may show right ventricular hypertrophy and right axis deviation;
echocardiogram diagnostic (older children may require transesophageal echo).
<u>Natural history</u>: Untreated lesions can lead to pulmonary HTN & CHF by 20-30 yrs.
Spontaneous closure rates by 3 yrs old of secundum ASD (if detected < 3 mo old)

<3 mm	3-8 mm	>8 mm
Approaching 100%	75-80%	Rare spontaneous closure

<u>Treatment</u>: Close for CHF, persistent lung disease, or signs of pulmonary HTN.
If ASD still present at 3-4 years of age, catheter device closure (ASD <20 mm and
adequate rim of surrounding tissue) or surgical repair recommended.

Circulation 1994;90:2180-8

ANTIBIOTIC PROPHYLAXIS FOR BACTERIAL ENDOCARDITIS

Limited to dental, oral, respiratory tract, skin, or musculoskeletal procedures in
patients at highest risk: Prosthetic heart valve, prior infective endocarditis,
valvulopathy after cardiac transplantation or cardiac repair, or many types of
congenital heart disease.
All regimens are single doses, administered 30-60 minutes prior to procedure.

Standard regimen	amoxicillin 50 mg/kg (max 2 g) PO
Unable to take oral medications	ampicillin 50 mg/kg (max 2 g) IV/IM; or ceftriaxone 50 mg/kg (max 1 g) IM/IV
Allergic to penicillin	clindamycin 20 mg/kg (max 600 mg) PO; or cephalexin† 50 mg/kg (max 2 g) PO; or azithromycin or clarithromycin 15 mg/kg (max 500mg) PO
Allergic to penicillin and unable to take oral medications	clindamycin 20 mg/kg (max 600 mg) IV/IM; or cefazolin† or ceftriaxone† 50 mg/kg (max 1 g) IV/IM

*For additional details see the 2007 American Heart Association guidelines at http://www.americanheart.org.
Prophylaxis is no longer recommended for genitourinary or gastrointestinal tract procedures.
†Avoid cephalosporins if prior penicillin-associated anaphylaxis, angioedema, or urticaria.

SYNCOPE & NEAR SYNCOPE

- *Syncope*: Transient loss of consciousness with resultant loss of muscle tone, or
- *Near syncope*: Transient alteration in mental status without unconscious period.

•Recent trauma or abnormal neurologic exam	Yes	Consider urgent head
•Palpitations, exercise induced, recurrent		CT, echo and/or ECG

No ↓

- **History and physical exam**: Assess hydration, blood pressure, medications
- **Past history**: Kawasaki disease, hypertension, congenital heart disease, palpitations
- **Family history**: Sudden cardiac death, early MI, Marfan's, long QT syndrome
- **Lab**: Blood glucose, pregnancy test, electrolytes, complete blood count
- **ECG**: Perform in all patients, unless clearly *not* cardiac. Consider Holter monitor

Differential diagnosis	History & Exam	Lab/radiology findings	Treatment
Neurocardiogenic (>50%)	•Prolonged standing •Prolonged fast •Emotional event •Rapid standing •Micturition •Defecation •Recent exercise	•Generally normal •Tilt-table test rarely used: (Sensitivity 26-80%, specificity 90%) •Consider Holter	•None •Medications rarely necessary, but may be helpful
Supraventricular tachycardia	•Palpitations •Normal exam	•ECG often normal •WPW: Delta wave •Holter monitor	•Cardiologist •Medication •Ablation
Long QT syndrome	•Recurrent syncope (cold water to face) •Previous "seizures"	•ECG: Long QTc •Screen family members	•β-blocker •Implantable defibrillator (ICD)
Aortic stenosis	•Exercise syncope •Systolic murmur	•ECG: LVH	•Valvuloplasty •Avoid exercise
Seizure (5-10%)	•Tonic-clonic •Post-ictal state	•Abnormal EEG and/or electrolytes	•Anti-epileptics •Neurologist
Migraine (5%)	•Headache, aura •Family history +	•Normal	•Identify triggers
Breath holding spell (2-5%)	•Toddler cries/holds breath until syncopal	•Normal	•Self-resolves by 5 years old
Hypertrophic cardiomyopathy (incidence=1:500)	•Syncope or chest pain during exercise •Family history +	•ECG: LVH •Echo diagnostic	•Exclusion from sports •ICD
Hyperventilation	•Anxiety, pain, etc	•↓ $PaCO_2$	•Relaxation

ECG=electrocardiogram, Echo=echocardiogram, EEG=electroencephalogram, Holter=Holter monitor, LVH=left ventricular hypertrophy, MI=myocardial infarction, WPW=Wolff-Parkinson-White syndrome

Circulation. 2006 Jan 17;113(2):316

ACNE

TYPES & CHARACTERISTICS OF ACNE

TYPE	CHARACTERISTICS
Comedonal	Whiteheads and/or blackheads
Inflammatory:	
Papulopustular	Papules and/ or pustules; most are < 5 mm in diameter.
Nodulocystic	**Nodules:** Pink/ purple, tender, deep, >5 mm. **Cysts:** Deeper than nodules, may be pink; ↑ scarring.
Cosmetic	Using comedogenic makeup, oils, lotions, cocoa butter, balms, pomades
Drug Induced	Steroids, cyclosporin A, isoniazid, rifampin, phenytoin, carbamazepine, lithium
Occupational	Exposure to mineral oil, tar, petroleum, hydrocarbons
Acne Conglobata	Severe, scarring, nodulocystic acne; involves face, chest, & back; usually white males starting in teen years.
Acne Fulminans	Abrupt onset of severe cystic acne progressing to ulcerated nodules; associated with fever, leukocytosis, arthralgias.
Tropical Acne	Papulopustular lesions on back/ buttocks in hot, humid weather or under occlusive clothing (football pads, backpacks).

DIFFERENTIAL DIAGNOSIS:
▶ Seborrhea, folliculitis, tinea barbae, rosacea, steroid abuse, adenoma sebaceum (tuberous sclerosis), perioral dermatitis

TREATMENT: ▶ Best results from using combination of therapies.
▶ Generally, acne may worsen before it improves (once treatment initiated).
▶ Try one agent for at least 3 months before switching, unless side effects present.
▶ All patients should be advised to avoid sun exposure or use sunscreen; many medications can ↑ photosensitivity.
▶ Consider hormonal therapy for women, especially if signs of hyperandrogenism.

Type of Acne	1st Line Treatment	2nd Line Treatment
Mild Comedonal	Benzoyl peroxide (BPO) or topical retinoid	Both benzoyl peroxide and topical retinoid
Mild Inflammatory	BPO + topical antibiotic	Add topical retinoid, consider oral antibiotics.
Moderate-Severe Comedonal	Topical retinoid	Increase potency of retinoid, add BPO.
Moderate-Severe Inflammatory	BPO + topical antibiotics ± oral antibiotics	All 3 topical agents and add oral antibiotics.
Nodulocystic	Systemic antibiotics ± BPO, topical retinoid	Isotretinoin

ACNE

Drug	How supplied & Brand names	Other
Benzoyl peroxide (BPO)	Start once daily, ↑ to bid if needed •Gel: 2.5%, 5%, 10% (Benzac AC, PanOxyl AQ) •Liquid: 2.5%, 5%, 10% (Benzac AC wash) •Cream 2.5%, 5%, 10% (Neutrogena On-the-Spot)	Side effects: skin irritation, peeling, dryness; Pregnancy category C Can bleach clothes.
Tretinoin (Retinoid)	•Cream: 0.025%, 0.05%, 0.1% (Retin-A, Altinac) •Gel: 0.01%, 0.025% (Retin-A, Avita), 0.04%, 0.1% (Retin-A Micro) •Liquid: 0.05% (cream & micro gel less irritating)	Use pea size amount to cover whole face. Use nightly. Skin irritation, peeling, photosensitivity.
Adapalene (Retinoid)	•1% gel, cream, pledgets, solution (Differin)	Pregnancy category C.
Tazarotene (Retinoid)	•Gel: 0.05%, 0.1% (Tazorac) •Cream: 0.05%, 0.1% (Tazorac)	Pregnancy category X.
Topical antibiotics	•Erythromycin 2% solution, gel, pledget daily-bid •Clindamycin 1% solution, gel, pledget; (Cleocin T, Clindagel) daily- bid	Avoid clindamycin in inflammatory bowel disease patients.
Topical antibiotics + BPO	•1% clindamycin/ 5% BPO (Duac Gel) •1% clindamycin/ 5% BPO (BenzaClin Gel) •3% erythromycin/ 5% BPO (Benzamycin)	Use daily to bid.
Topical antibiotics + Tretinoin	•1.2% clindamycin/ 0.025% tretinoin (Ziana Gel)	
Systemic antibiotics†	•Tetracycline 250-1500 mg/ day •Doxycycline 50-200 mg/ day •Minocycline 50-200 mg/ day	GI upset, esophageal ulcer, pigmentation changes.
Isotretinoin	•0.5-1 mg/kg/day divided BID for 15-20 weeks; 10, 20, 40 mg capsules (Accutane, Sotret, Amnesteem, Claravis) •Side effects: Dry mouth, ↓ night vision, photosensitivity; can affect all organ systems.	Start 2 reliable forms of contraception 1 month before starting isotretinoin. Obtain written consent. Monthly pregnancy test, CBC, LFT's, lipids.
Hormonal therapy	•Oral contraceptive pills (OCP): Yasmin, Ortho Tri-cyclen, Estrostep •Spironolactone: 50-200 mg/ day	Allow 3-6 months for benefit Pregnancy category X; Use with OCP's.

GI: Gastrointestinal; LFT's: Liver Function Test   †Use only in patients > 8 years old

ECZEMA

PHASES OF ECZEMA

Age	Phase	Characteristics
< 2 years	Infantile	Cheeks, face, scalp. Red papules/ vesicles; pruritus. May be at higher risk of developing asthma later in life.
2- teens	Childhood	Hands, feet, wrists, ankles, antecubital/popliteal fossae papules/ lichenified plaques.
After puberty	Adult	Flexural folds, face, hands, feet. Red, scaling papules or lichenified plaques.

RISK FACTORS: + Family history of eczema or other atopic diseases (asthma/ allergies), ↑ food specific IgE (~1/3 of kids with eczema, though in most patients taking food out of diet will not decrease flares; extensively hydrolyzed casein formula may ↓eczema in the first year of life in high-risk kids), exposure to environmental allergens (dust, mites).

OTHER FORMS:
▶ *Nummular*: Circular patches (can look like granuloma annulare)
▶ *Dyshidrotic*: Small deep vesicles in clusters on palms, soles, lateral fingers→ lichenification/ fissuring.

DIFFERNTIAL DIAGNOSIS: Contact dermatitis, tinea corporis, psoriasis, scabies. Rare: Langerhans cell histiocytosis, vitamin deficiency, cutaneous T-cell lymphoma

TREATMENT: ▶ DAILY: Mild water temperatures, unscented or no soap, emollient to wet skin, avoid irritants such as perfumes/ dyes/ fabric softeners, irritant clothing.
▶ FLARES:
1) *Topical medications*: <u>Steroid creams</u>: May use ↑potency for immediate relief and ↓ potency for maintenance. Consider <u>calcineurin inhibitors</u> (ie. tacrolimus) for kids > 2 years. <u>Topical antibiotics</u> + topical steroid may result in greater improvement. <u>Atopiclair</u> (glycyrrhetinic acid (2%) and hyaluronic acid) nonsteroidal cream recently FDA approved, no limit on duration or age of use.
2) *Antibiotics* (topical if mild/ localized, oral if more severe/ widespread) if signs of superinfection; if recurrent infections, consider topical antiseptics (triclosan/ chlorhexidine) 1-3 times/ week, antibacterial soaps (Lever 2000®), chlorine (1 tsp/gallon) baths if tolerated (may help decrease colonization with *Staph aureus*).
▶ Anti-pruritic medications: Diphenhydramine, hydroxyzine.
▶ Refer to dermatology if unclear diagnosis or unresponsive to treatment. Short course systemic steroids or ultraviolet light therapy sometimes indicated.

COMPLICATIONS
▶ Herpes simplex virus: Use oral acyclovir or valacyclovir, continue eczema treatment. Systemic/ diffuse disease (eczema herpeticum) can be life-threatening, requiring hospitalization.
▶ Other skin infections, especially *Staph aureus*.
▶ Long term use of topical steroids can cause hypopigmentation, skin atrophy, systemic absorption, hypothalamic-pituitary axis suppression (↑ with higher potency steroids, use on high body surface area, or if occlusive dressing used).

Boguniewicz M - *Immunol Allergy Clin North Am* - 01-MAY-2005;25(2): 333-51

ECZEMA CONTINUED

TOPICAL ANTIINFLAMMATORIES

Avoid mucous membranes/eyes. Wash hands after applying.

Low-topical steroids (use in infants; facial, mild-moderate eczema)	•**Very Low Potency: hydrocortisone (HC)** 0.5% cream/ ointment; 1% cream, ointment
	•**Low Potency: HC** 2.5% cream, ointment **alclometasone dipropionate** (*Aclovate*) 0.05% cream, ointment **fluocinolone acetonide** (*Synalar* cream 0.01%) **triamcinolone acetonide (TAC)** 0.025%
Mid-potency topical steroids (listed in order of increasing potency; use for moderate to severe eczema, especially older children. Avoid using on face/ periorbital area)	•**MID: hydrocortisone valerate** 0.2% cream, ointment **betamethasone valerate** 0.1% cream **fluocinolone acetonide** (*Synalar*) 0.025% cream **fluticasone propionate** (*Cutivate*) 0.05% cream **fluocinolone acetonide** (*Derma-Smoothe* oil) 0.01% **mometasone furoate** (*Elocon*) 0.1% cream **TAC** (*Kenalog*) 0.1% cream
	•**UPPER: TAC** 0.1% ointment, **TAC** 0.5% cream **fluticasone propionate** (*Cutivate*) 0.005% ointment **betamethasone dipropionate** 0.05%
High-potency topical steroids (consult dermatologist)	**desoximetasone** (*Topicort*) 0.25% cream, ointment **mometasone furoate** (*Elocon*) 0.1% ointment **fluocinonide** (*Lidex*) 0.05% ointment, cream, gel
Calcineurin inhibitors (very useful on face; approved for ≥2 yrs old)	**tacrolimus ointment** (*Protopic*) 0.03%, 0.1% **pimecrolimus** (*Elidel*) 1%: Less local side effects than topical steroids. Use BID for short periods of time.
Topical Nonsteroidal	**Atopiclair** (glycyrrhetinic acid/ hyaluronic acid) BID

*mometasone and fluticasone may have fewer side effects including skin atrophy. Ointments often more potent than cream/ lotion; generally apply BID for up to 1 week.

ANTIPRURITIC MEDICATIONS: (sedating antihistamines)

Diphenhydramine	2-4 mg/kg/day in 4 divided doses (max 50 mg/dose); 12.5 mg/ 5 mL elixir, syrup, liquid; 12.5 mg chew & 25, 50 mg tabs
Hydroxyzine (*Atarax, Vistaril*)	2 mg/kg/day divided every 6-8 hours. Syrup: 10 mg/5 mL; suspension: 25 mg/5 mL; tabs: 10, 25, 50,100 mg.

ANTI-INFECTIVE AGENTS

Cephalexin	50 mg/kg/d qid; 125 mg or 250 mg/5 mL; tabs: 250, 500 mg
Trimethoprim-sulfamethoxazole	6-12 mg/kg/d TMP bid; 40 mg/ 5 mL susp; 80 mg tabs; DS 160 mg tabs (useful for methicillin-resistant *Staph Aureus*)
Mupirocin	2% cream/ ointment tid for 5-10 days.
Acyclovir	*Herpes simplex:* 1000 mg/day 3-5 doses x 7-14 days (max: 80 mg/kg/day) 200 mg/5 ml, tabs: 400 mg, 800 mg; *Varicella:* 20 mg/kg/dose (max 800 mg/dose) qid x 5 d (start by 24 hr)

DIAPER RASH

Dermatitis	Clinical findings	Treatment
Irritant (contact)	•Exposure to urine & stool •Spares inguinal area/folds •Can be peri-anal if due to diarrhea •Secondary infection common	•Expedite diaper changes •Allow area to air dry •Zinc oxide or petrolatum barrier each diaper change •Avoid talcum powder
Candidal	•Beefy red, confluent, wet •Peripheral oval "satellite" papules •Involves inguinal area/folds	•Miconazole 0.25% oint •Nystatin •Clotrimazole 1% cream
Seborrhea	•Patchy or focal greasy, scaly, red, papules (consider immune problem if FTT & chronic diarrhea)	•Dry folds completely •Hydrocortisone 1% bid-qid may improve lesions
Scabies	•Pruritic, papulonodular, crusted •May have pustules •Secondary impetigo common	•Permethrin 5% x 8-14 hrs •Treat household contacts
Perianal Strep	•Shiny red, tender, sharp-margins •Itching, painful defecation	•Antibiotics (penicillin) •Inpatient if neonate, toxic
Staph Aureus	•Impetigo (honey colored crust) or bullae	•Anti-staphylococcal antibiotics
Psoriasis	•Bright red, well demarcated scaly plaques unresponsive to treatment •Entire perineal area, skin folds	•Diagnosis often by biopsy •Consult dermatologist
Langerhans cell histiocytosis	•Crusted, scaling lesions •Central red-brown purpuric papules •Involves scalp, axilla, behind ear	•Biopsy proven diagnosis •Extensive evaluation to determine severity, extent of systemic involvement

FTT=failure to thrive, oint=ointment

CONTACT DERMATITIS

	Causes	Treatment
Irritant	•Lip-licking/thumb sucking xerosis •Chemical irritation in diaper area	•Moisturizer to restore skin barrier •Remove offending stimulus
Allergic	•Poison ivy/oak •Nickel •Cosmetics •Neomycin	•Mild symptoms: Low-medium potency topical steroid x 2-3 weeks for <10% body surface area (triamcinolone 0.1% oint to extremities, hydrocortisone for face, skin folds) •Severe symptoms: Systemic corticosteroids: 1-2 mg/kg/day in single morning dose. Response within 7 days. Taper over 1-2 wks to prevent rebound flare. Add antihistamine. •Consider using domeboro's solution soaks for vesicles, crusting of poison ivy/oak.

	SKIN INFECTIONS - 1		
Infection	**Symptoms**	**Treatment**	**How Supplied**
Scabies	Itching, ↑ at night. Creases hands/ feet/ axilla, diaper area. Papules, vesicles, tracking. May itch for 2-4 weeks after treated.	Treat all close contacts (unless pregnant) Wash clothes/ bedding in hot water after treated. Permethrin 5% neck down overnight. Repeat in 1 week (unless pregnant, or < 2 months old)	Permethrin 5% cream (Elimite, Acticin) Pregnancy category B, use caution in pregnant or breastfeeding women and infants < 2 months. May use topical steroids for relief of itching.
Lice	Itching scalp, eggs/ lice on scalp	Permethrin 90% effective. Conditioner/ olive oil then comb BID x 1 week after last louse noted (1/3 cure); Shaving head not effective. Wash bedding in hot water.	Permethrin liquid 1% (crème rinse) for 10 minutes, then rinse. Repeat in 1 week. If persist, may use permethrin 5% under shower cap overnight. Louse resistance: malathion 0.5% lotion x 8-12 hours.
Impetigo	Honey colored crust (Staph or Strep) or bullae (bullous impetigo= S. Aureus); Up to 50% of S. Aureus is methicillin resistant.	Mupirocin topically or systemic antibiotics if bullous/ febrile/ extensive.	> 2 months: Mupirocin (Bactroban) 2% cream or ointment TID x 5-14 days. For systemic treatment, cephalexin, trimethoprim-sulfamethoxazole, or clindamycin.
Abscess	Red, swollen, tender. Often fluctuant or with "head" or spontaneously draining. ± Associated cellulitis/ systemic symptoms.	Incision and drainage if fluctuant/ head. Treat with trimethoprim sulfamethoxazole or clindamycin if associated cellulitis/ systemic symptoms.	Trimethoprim/ sulfamethoxazole 6-12 mg/kg trimethoprim (TMP) component/day divided Q 12 hours (40mg TMP/ 5 mL suspension). Clindamycin 10-25 mg/kg/ day PO divided tid-qid (oral solution 75mg/ 5mL).

SKIN INFECTIONS - 2

Infection	Symptoms	Work-up / Treatment	Treatment
Cellulitis	Erythema, warmth, swelling, pain; usually Group A or B Strep, ?Staph (MRSA & MSSA). Puncture wound/hot tub : Pseudomonas; Human bite: anaerobes, strep pyogenes; cat/dog bite: pasteurella	Consider CBC, blood culture, C-reactive protein; mild infections treated with oral cephalexin, trimethoprim sulfamethoxazole, or clindamycin and monitor closely; if febrile, toxic, infant or severe infection, admit for IV antibiotics.	Cephalexin: 50 mg/kg/day divided qid (max 500 po qid). Trimethoprim/ sulfamethoxazole 6-12 mg/kg trimethoprim (TMP) component/ day divided q 12 hrs. (suspension: 40mg TMP/ 5 mL; tablet 80 mg TMP; DS 160mg)
Preseptal vs Orbital Cellulitis	Preseptal: around eye but no proptosis, normal extraocular movements, normal vision. Orbital cellulitis is an ophthalmologic emergency. Most commonly caused by Staph, Strep, H. Flu.	Consider CBC, c-reactive protein, blood culture; if afebrile and preseptal cellulitis may treat with cephalexin, amoxicillin- clavulanate or trimethoprim-sulfamethoxazole; close followup warranted. Admit orbital cellulitis, consult ophtho	Cephalexin & trimethoprim-sulfamethoxazole dosing as above.
Perianal cellulitis	Group A streptococcus	Penicillin V, cephalexin, erythromycin.	Penicillin V 25-50 mg/kg/ day qid; cephalexin 50 mg/ kg/ day qid erythromycin 40 mg/kg/ day qid
Erysipelas	Rapid onset, fever, superficial shiny erythema with elevated borders; usually lower extremities.	Primary organism is strep pyogenes.	Penicillin, cephalexin; admit if toxic or febrile.
Furuncle, Carbuncle, Folliculitis	Inflammation at hair follicles; multiple lesions are usually carbuncles; Usually caused by Staph aureus.	Warm compress, incision & drainage if fluctuant; antibacterial washes; topical clindamycin or mupirocin.	Systemic antibiotics for carbuncles or cellulitis with systemic symptoms.

Primary Care: Clinics in Office Practice 2006: 33(3) ; Infect Dis Clin North Am 2006 : 20 (4) pp. 759-772

			SKIN INFECTIONS - 3
Infection	Symptoms	Work-up / Treatment	Treatment
Tinea Corporis	Round scaling plaque, raised edge, central clearing; may see papules, vesicles, bullae.	*Topical:* miconazole, clotrimazole, ketoconazole cream, terbinafine cream. *Systemic:* For patients with chronic, recurrent infections, or if immune compromised. Griseofulvin microsize 10-20 mg/kg po daily (or ultramicrosize 5-10 mg/kg/day)	rash clears (usually minimum 4 weeks of treatment). Systemic: Griseofulvin: kids > 2 yrs. Should be taken with fatty meal x 2-4 weeks. (microsize: 125mg/ 5 mL or tablets 250mg, 500 mg). ultramicrosize: 125mg, 165mg).
Onychomycosis	Discoloration and peeling of nails; Differential diagnosis: nail psoriasis, lichen planus; culture prior to starting oral treatment.	Ciclopirox (Penlac Nail Lacquer) for superficial; Systemic: Terbinafine* orally, itraconazole*, griseofulvin can be considered but has poor success rate and requires prolonged course.	Terbinafine (250 mg tabs) 3-6 mg/kg/day po (fingernails: 6 weeks, toenails: 12 weeks); Itraconazole** 1wk/ month x 2-3 months. (< 20 kg: 5 mg/kg/day; 20-40 kg: 100 mg/ day; 40-50 kg: 200 mg/ day, > 50 kg: 200 mg bid)
Tinea Capitis	Patchy scaling, alopecia, broken hairs ("black dot"), postauricular adenopathy, kerion (boggy inflammatory mass)	Griseofulvin microsize 10-20 mg/kg/day po or ultramicrosize 5-10 mg/kg/day; selenium sulfide shampoo 1-2.5% decreases fungal shedding. Kerion: add prednisone 1-2 mg/kg/d x 2 weeks. Culture before starting treatment.	Griseofulvin for kids > 2 years old. Treat x 6-8 weeks; continue 2 weeks beyond resolution. Liver function tests if on prolonged therapy (> 8 weeks) or symptoms.

* Itraconazole and terbinafine not approved for use in kids for this indication; safety and efficacy not determined. Exercise caution and monitor renal/ hepatic/ cardiac function.
Dermatol Clin - 01-APR-2007; 25(2): 165-83; Lexi Comp's Pediatric Dosage Handbook; Dermatol Clin - 01-JUL-2006; 24(3): 355-63.

VIRAL EXANTHEMS - 1

Virus/Syndrome	Rash	Associated Symptoms	Incubation/ Spread	Complications/ Other
Paramyxovirus (Measles, Rubeola)	Begins at head, spreads to chest/ abdomen, extremities; red/ violaceous macules which may coalesce; lasts 5-7 days	Prodrome of fever, cough, coryza, conjunctivitis; gray papules on buccal mucosa 1-2 days before exanthem appears.	Increased risk if not immunized or recent foreign travel; spread by respiratory droplets; contagious 4 days before and after rash; 14 days incubation	Pneumonia, myocarditis, encephalitis, subacute sclerosing panencephalitis (SSPE)
Parvovirus B19 ("Slapped Cheeks", Fifth Disease)	Begins at face with bright red cheeks; erythematous rash ("lacy") at trunk/ extremities later; increased rash with heat (i.e. after bath)	Occasional fever, cold symptoms; 10% have joint pain.	Spread by respiratory droplets. 30% maternal-fetal transmission if mom infected. Contagious until exanthem appears; lifelong immunity	Fetal infection may result in hydrops (3%) or miscarriage (increased risk in 2nd trimester). Increased risk of aplastic crisis in people with hemolytic anemia.
Rubella (German Measles)	Pink maculopapular rash spreads from head to feet. Clears within 72 hours.	Soft palate red spots; may see mild fever, coryza, adenopathy, arthritis	Incubation 2-3 weeks; contagious 3 days before/ after rash appears	Fetal infection (congenital rubella syndrome); encephalitis, arthritis
Varicella (Chickenpox)	Crops of papules→ vesicles→crusting (all stages present at once); starts at trunk and spreads; pruritic/ painful	Mild systemic symptoms/ fever; older patients have more severe symptoms; May also see vesicles on mucous membranes.	Contagious 3 days before rash until all lesions are crusted; 14 days incubation; acyclovir 80 mg/ kg/ day PO (max 3200 mg) x 5 days for kids > 12 yrs old (IV if immunocompromised)	Skin infections, keratitis pneumonia, encephalitis, hepatitis, myocarditis; fetal complications [Varicella Zoster Immune Globulin (VZIG) for nonimmune pregnant women]

| | | | VIRAL EXANTHEMS - 2 |
Virus/Syndrome	Rash	Associated Symptoms	Incubation/Spread	Complications/Other
Human Herpes Virus 6 or 7 (*Roseola*)	Maculopapular rash starts at trunk with abrupt defervescence.	Kids 6-36 months; high fever for 3-5 days without other symptoms	Incubation 10 days; usually transmitted by asymptomatic contact	Febrile seizures seen in 10% of infected kids.
Coxsackie A16 / enterovirus 71 (*Hand-Foot-Mouth*)	Vesicles at palms/soles in about 65% of those infected.	Low grade fever, malaise, may have upper respiratory symptoms	Incubation 3-6 days; contagious for ≥ 1 week.	Beware of dehydration.
Epstein-Barr Virus (*EBV; mononucleosis*)	5-10% have rash; can be maculopapular, petechial, scarlatiniform, urticarial	Fever, pharyngitis, adenopathy, splenomegaly	Incubation 1-2 months; Life-long intermittent viral shedding.	May get rash if treated with amoxicillin/ ampicillin; splenic rupture, pneumonia, meningitis.
Herpes Simplex Virus 1 (HSV) (*herpetic gingivostomatitis*)	Thick-walled vesicles on erythematous base, usually at lips or fingers	>90% of primary HSV-1 infections are asymptomatic; fever, adenopathy possible	Incubation 2 days-2 weeks. Can shed virus for ≥1 week. Spread by contact with secretions.	Eczema herpeticum, encephalitis, keratoconjunctivitis.
Herpes Zoster	Macules lead to papules lead to vesicles in dermatomal distribution	± fever, adenopathy, pain at dermatome	2 week incubation; spread by direct contact with lesions.	Postherpetic neuralgia, dissemination if immunocompromised
Gianotti Crosti Syndrome (*Papular Acrodermatitis of Childhood*)	Pink papulovesicles at cheeks, extensor surface of extremities, buttocks; symmetric; coalesce	±prodrome of upper respiratory infection, pharyngitis, diarrhea, lymphadenopathy	Caused by many possible viruses including hepatitis A or B, EBV, HSV, and post vaccination	Rash may last up to 2 months; other complications depend on causative virus.

VASCULAR SKIN LESIONS

	Description	Natural history / Treatment	Associated Problems
Hemangioma	• Dome-shaped, superficial, deep (subcutaneous or dermal), or visceral (liver, brain, colon) conglomeration of abnormal blood vessels • Present in 2-5% neonates • F:M = 3:1	• Expand for 6-10 months, then involute over next several years • Possible residual atrophy, wrinkling, hypopigmentation, redundant skin, telangiectasia • 5-10% ulcerate during growth (treat to prevent scarring) • Small lesions rarely need treatment. Consider pulsed dye laser, glucocorticoids (potent topical, oral, or injected) for large lesions or those in special sites (peri-orbital)	• Lip, nasal, pre-auricular, or chin lesions may predict tracheal or oropharyngeal lesions and may result in disfigurement. Refer to dermatologist. • Diffuse neonatal hemangiomatosis: Rare condition associated with multiple cutaneous and visceral hemangiomas. Can have high-output cardiac failure, respiratory failure, obstructive jaundice and may lead to death. • Peri-orbital: Refer to ophthalmology • Sacral lesions: Rare tethered cord, dysraphism • PHACE syndrome: Posterior fossa anomaly (Dandy-Walker cyst), hemangioma (large, facial, >1 dermatome), arterial anomalies, coarctation of the aorta, eye anomalies.
Port-wine stain	• Macular, sharp borders, pink-purple, varying size	• Pink at birth, darken with age, occasional bleeding, laser treatment may be effective	• Sturge-Weber: 8% lesions in cranial nerve V distribution associated with glaucoma, seizure • Overgrowth of extremity from large lesions
Cystic hygroma	• Cavernous lymphatic malformation on face, trunk	• Large, often multilocular, deep, rubbery nodules, may develop internal bleeding	• Surgery very difficult, often reaccumulate. • Intralesional sclerosing agents if disfiguring • Posterior neck lesions may be associated with Turner syndrome.
Pyogenic granuloma	• Small, red, pedunculated mass on face, arms, hands • Fragile and friable	• Grow rapidly • Trauma leads to bleeding. • Silver nitrate small lesions	• Larger lesions may need shave excision with cautery to base to prevent recurrence.

HYPOPIGMENTED SKIN LESIONS

	Description	Natural history	Associated problems / Treatment
Vitiligo	• Sharp-bordered, flat, patchy, depigmentation. • Generalized symmetric vs. segmental • Often acral, perioral/facial	• 50% present <18 yrs old • Remission 10-20% • Slowly progressive	• Rarely associated with endocrinopathies (diabetes, hypothyroidism, Addison's disease) • Topical treatment with steroids or tacrolimus • Narrow band ultraviolet B phototherapy for generalized disease: 50% of patients get 75% repigmentation.
Hypopigmented whorls	• Sharp hypopigmentation lines on trunk, extremities	• Present at birth, often persists to adulthood	• Hypomelanosis of Ito: Equal ♀:♂, mental retardation, seizures, microcephaly, hypotonia
Pityriasis alba	• Oval, flat, scaly patches on face, extensor arms, trunk	• ~30% children affected • Lesions repigment in months, but condition lasts several years	• Emollients +/- hydrocortisone 1% • Differentiate from tinea versicolor with KOH stain
Oculocutaneous albinism	• Complete or partial lack of pigment in hair, skin, eyes	• Autosomal recessive	• Adequate skin protection from ultraviolet light (clothing, sunscreen) to prevent skin cancer • Nystagmus, strabismus, decreased visual acuity
Partial albinism (piebaldism)	• Forehead, knees, elbows, scalp (white forelock), trunk	• Autosomal dominant	• Differentiate from vitiligo, which is progressive • May respond to phototherapy or surgery
Incontinentia pigmenti	• X-linked dominant, seen only in females. • 4 stages: Vesicular (neonate), linear verrucous lesions (< 1 yr old), hyperpigmented swirls (childhood), fade to hypopigmented lesions by adolescence.		• Mental retardation, seizures, microcephaly, ocular and skeletal anomalies occur occasionally • 90% have dental anomalies (delayed eruption)
Ash leaf macules	• White, sharp borders, leaf-shaped noted at birth, or shortly after, on trunk or extremities. Use Wood's lamp.		• Tuberous sclerosis (See neurocutaneous disorders pp. 146)

POLYCYSTIC OVARIAN SYNDROME (PCOS)

- **Pathogenesis**: Androgen excess resulting in chronic ovarian dysfunction. Exact mechanism unknown, though central obesity and insulin resistance likely key.
- **Prevalence**: 4-10% of women, onset in adolescence. Premature pubarche may be an early sign of PCOS.

Diagnosis: No definitive criteria exist. 2 of 3 below criteria suggest PCOS
Irregular menses: Anovulation or oligo-ovulation leads to oligo or amenorrhea
Hyperandrogenism: Clinical (hirsutism, acne, alopecia) or by lab analysis
Polycystic ovaries: Ultrasound (US): Ovaries >10cm^3, >12 follicles 2-9 mm, ↑echogenicity
*Adolescents have anovulation (50% of all cycles) in 1st 2-3 yrs after menarche *and* cystic ovaries on ultrasound, so hyperandrogenism crucial to diagnosis.

Differential diagnosis: Late-onset congenital adrenal hyperplasia, androgen secreting tumors, hyperprolactinemia, Cushing's syndrome, iatrogenic
Associated findings: Premature adrenarche or pubarche, acanthosis nigricans, obesity, seborrhea, hyperhidrosis

Lab Analysis: Total testosterone: Normal: 70-90 ng/dL; PCOS: 90-150 ng/dL; Androgen secreting tumor: >200 ng/dL.

- Pelvic US: Transvaginal more sensitive, not recommended in virginal patients.
- DHEAS: Elevated levels in adrenal disorders (usually leads to rapid virilization).
- Extended work-up to rule out other causes includes thyroid function, prolactin, 8 a.m. cortisol and 17-hydroxyprogesterone levels.
- Once diagnosis confirmed, check insulin, lipid levels, glucose tolerance test.

Potential Long-term Complications

•Infertility: Improved by combined oral contraceptives and metformin
•Obesity (50% of patients): ↑ risk of obstructive sleep apnea syndrome
•Metabolic syndrome: Insulin resistance →impaired glucose tolerance
•Coronary artery disease: ↑risk due to hyperlipidemia and insulin resistance
•Endometrial hyperplasia/carcinoma: Chronic anovulation = ↑estrogen exposure

TREATMENT

1. Weight loss via ↓caloric intake & ↑exercise usually unsuccessful.
2. *Menstrual irregularity:* Combined (estrogen + progestin) oral contraceptive (COC). Progestins norgestimate & drospirenone have ↓androgenic effects (↓hirsutism, acne). Recheck symptoms and androgen levels at 3 months. If androgens still high, consider alternate diagnosis. If improved, continue COC for five years post-menarche. 2nd line agents for menstrual irregularity include progestin alone, low-dose nightly glucocorticoid therapy, or gonadotropin releasing hormone agonist (GnRH).
3. Metformin (↓insulin,↑ovulation): Used for metabolic syndrome and obesity. Start 500 mg nightly meal, increase by 500 mg weekly to max 2000 mg/day. Causes significant nausea and diarrhea. Check yearly creatinine, liver enzymes.
4. Spironolactone (100–200 mg/day divided bid): Effective for hirsutism. Use with COC to prevent pregnancy & fetal teratogenicity and irregular bleeding.
5. Topical eflornithine hydrochloride cream ↓facial hair growth in 6-8 weeks.

DHEAS=Dehydroepiandrosterone;   Obstet Gynecol 2002; 100(6):1389-402, *Hum Reprod* 2004; 19(1):41-725.

TYPE 1 DIABETES MELLITUS IN CHILDREN (T1DM)

Diagnosis: Affects 170/100,000 kids <19 yrs old, mean onset 8-12 yrs, 1:1 ♂:♀
1) Random/casual blood glucose (BG) >200mg/dL (11.1 mmol/L) + symptoms, or
2) Fasting blood glucose >126 mg/dL (7 mmol/L), or
3) 2 hr blood glucose ≥ 200 mg/dL after 75 gram (g) oral glucose tolerance test

Pathophysiology:

	Immune mediated pancreatic beta cell destruction	
Hyperglycemia	**Insulin deficiency**	Ketosis
Polyuria, polydipsia, nocturia, weight loss, malaise		Nausea, vomiting
	Dehydration, acidosis, altered mental status	

New Onset T1DM: If no evidence of acidosis at diagnosis, inpatient or outpatient intensive education at specialty center equally effective, without ↑risk to patient.
Cochrane Database of Systematic Reviews 2007, Issue 2. Art. No.: CD004099

TOTAL DAILY INSULIN DOSE (TDD)

40-50% long-acting insulin, 50-60% short-acting insulin
•Pre-adolescents: 0.5-0.75 units/kg/day •Adolescents: 0.75 – 1 unit/kg/day
"Honeymoon" period: Residual endogenous insulin decreases exogenous needs

- **Basal-bolus technique**: Patient must be taught to count carbohydrates (carb).
  - Long-acting insulin for basal needs given once or twice daily
  - Rapid-acting insulin 5-15 minutes before meals (consider giving "picky eaters" insulin *after* eating to limit hypoglycemic risk)   *Diabetes Care*. 1999 Jan;22(1):133-6
  - Meal insulin: carb ratio may vary by age from 1:30 in children to 1:5 in adolescents (↑insulin resistance, particularly in a.m. from ↑growth hormone)
- **Insulin pump**: Continuous rapid-acting insulin (basal) via a pump, bolus for meals.

Insulin type	Name	Onset (hrs)	Peak (hrs)	Duration (hrs)	Peak low BG risk
Rapid-acting	lispro or aspart	5-10 min	0.5-2	2-3	2-3 hrs
Fast-acting	regular	0.5-1	2-5	6-8	3-7 hrs
Intermediate-acting	NPH (isophane) or lente	1-3	5-8	8-18	4-16 hrs
Long-acting	ultralente	3-4	8-15	22-26	8-18 hrs
Very long-acting	glargine (*Lantus*) or detemir	1.5-4	None	20-24	5-10 hrs

*Mixed insulin solutions (70/30) should *not be used* for management of children unless significant barriers to diabetic control exist. These preparations *do not* take into account variable glucose levels, exercise or meal volumes.

CORRECTION DOSE

- Additional short-acting insulin to correct hyperglycemia (see table next page)
- **1800 rule**: 1800/TDD = expected drop in BG (mg/dL) by 1 unit rapid-acting insulin.
  - Do not give correction dose more than q2 hrs (or duration of given insulin used).
  - Consider half of correction dose at bedtime
  - Unless ill or ketotic, no correction overnight given risk of hypoglycemia.

TYPE 1 DIABETES MELLITUS (CONTINUED)

BLOOD GLUCOSE (BG) MONITORING

- Before meals, at bedtime and, for 1 week after changing basal insulin, at 2 a.m.
- 2-hour post-prandial BG results used to adjust rapid-acting insulin:carb ratio.
- Overnight BG & multi-day trends useful in adjusting basal insulin.
- *Sick-day*: Increase BG & ketone monitoring as hypo & hyperglycemia common. Insulin needs generally ↑, but may ↓while ill. Poor PO intake=↑risk hypoglycemia.

T1DM THERAPY GOALS: Limit BG fluctuations by pairing insulin with needs.

Age	Hemoglobin A1C	Bedtime glucose	Pre-meal glucose
< 6 years old	7.5-8.5%	110-200 mg/dL	100-180 mg/dL
6-12 years old	≤8%	100-180 mg/dL	90-180 mg/dL
13-19 years old	≤7.5%	90-150 mg/dL	90-130 mg/dL

Diabetic Ketoacidosis (DKA): pH < 7.3 or serum bicarbonate <16 mEq/L.
- ↑ risk of cerebral edema with more severe illness & younger children. ~30% new-onset T1DM have DKA.

Ketones: Check urine or serum ketones if BG >250 mg/dL x2, or if ill/emesis.
- If ketones present, consider correction dose and monitor for signs of DKA.

Hypoglycemia: Signs/symptoms: Irritability, headache, lethargy, hunger, tremor, sweating, palpitations, difficult to arouse, seizures. Infants have subtle symptoms.
- BG <70 or symptomatic: "15/15 rule"= eat 15 g rapidly absorbed carb (4 oz. juice), recheck BG in 15 mins. If next meal >30 mins away, add protein (peanut butter).
- Glucagon: <20 kg = 0.02-0.03 mg/kg or 0.5 mg IM/SQ q20 minutes as needed.
  >20 kg = 1 mg IM/SQ q20 minutes as needed *if unable to eat/drink*.

Diet: Goal ~50-55% carbs, 15-20% protein, 30% fat. Ok to eat >3 meals/day.

Exercise: ↑hypoglycemic risk during and after exercise (including overnight)
- Check BG q30 min during, q15 min after prolonged exercise *and* at 2 a.m.
- If on long-acting insulin, snack (15 g carb) prior to and every 30 minutes during prolonged exercise.
- Patients on insulin pump: ↓basal by 30-70% prior to exercise.

Adjunctive Therapy / Future Directions

- Continuous BG monitor: Detects nighttime low BG & hypoglycemic unawareness.
- Metformin (biguanide): Useful in pubertal children with severe insulin resistance.
- Pramlintide (*Amylin*): Injection. ↓gluconeogenesis & slows intestinal absorption of nutrients = ↓post-prandial hyperglycemia & HbA1c without hypoglycemia.
- Inhaled insulin: Trials encouraging in adolescents/adults. ↑patient satisfaction.

Long-term Considerations / Screening

Depression	25-33% prevalence; factor in poor compliance/recurrent DKA
Retinopathy	Age ≥10 and T1DM >3-5yrs: Annual ophthalmologic exam
Nephropathy	Age ≥10 and T1DM ≥5yrs: Annual microalbumin: creatinine. If abnormal, consult nephrology and consider ACE inhibitor. Blood pressure & lipid control crucial. Avoid smoking.
Thyroid disease	Thyroid stimulating hormone (TSH) at diagnosis and q1-2 yrs
Celiac disease	Screen at diagnosis, and every 3-5 years
Eating disorders	Consider in underweight patients or those with recurrent DKA.

Diabetes. 2005 Apr;54(4):1100-7J Clin Endocrinol Metab. 2007 Mar;92(3):815-6, Diabetes Care 28:186-212, 2005

PUBERTY

Tanner Stages (average age range)

	Tanner 1	Tanner 2	Tanner 3	Tanner 4	Tanner 5
Female Breast	Pre-adolescent	Breast bud (8-12 yrs)	Enlarged but no secondary mound (10-12 yrs)	Areola→ secondary mound (13 yrs, highly variable)	Mature breasts (12-19 yrs; variable)
Female Pubic Hair	Fine hair only	Sparse, pigmented, downy hair (9-12 yrs)	Darker, curlier, coarser hair	Adult pattern, lesser quantity; none at thighs	Adult pattern and amount, spread to thighs
Male Genitals	Pre-adolescent	↑ size scrotum / testis; Δ testis skin texture (11-13 yrs)	↑ penis length (some diameter)	Enlargement of all elements, darkened scrotal skin.	Adult size and shape.
Male Pubic Hair	Fine hair only	Pigmented downy hair	Darker, curly, coarse	Adult pattern, lesser quantity	Adult pattern/ quantity; thighs

▶ **Order of Puberty**:
- *Girls*: thelarche→adrenarche→menarche (2-3 years after thelarche); peak growth at 11-12 years;
- *Boys*: ↑testicle size→pubic hair→penile enlargement→face hair; peak growth at 13-14 years.

▶ **Factors that influence onset of puberty:** Race (African American usually earlier than Caucasian), genetics, adoption from developing to developed country, obesity.

PRECOCIOUS PUBERTY

▶ Defined as the early onset of sexual secondary sex characteristics. Boys ≤ 9 years old; girls ≤ 8 years old.

▶ 80% of cases of precocious puberty are central. 85% of central precocious puberty (CPP) in girls is idiopathic. 60% of boys with central precocious puberty have underlying pathology. 2% of girls age 6-8 with central precocious puberty had abnormal MRI; 20% of girls with central precocious puberty <6 had abnormal MRI.

PUBERTY – CLINICAL & LAB FINDINGS IN VARIOUS DISORDERS

Disorder	Signs	Bone age x-rays	LH*, FSH	Testosterone, estradiol
Central precocious puberty	↑ growth rate, ↑ testicle size (♂)	↑ Bone age (equals stage of pubertal development > chronological age)	Pubertal range (increased: LH> 0.3 IU/L*)	Pubertal range
Peripheral precocious puberty	↑ growth rate	↑ Bone age	Suppressed (prepubertal)	Increased
Congenital adrenal hyperplasia (CAH)	Normal testicle size (♂); pubic hair, body odor, acne	More advanced than expected in puberty	Normal	Variable
Premature thelarche†	Girls 6 months -8 years old, <2 years old most common; no ↑ growth rate	Normal bone age (equals chronological age)	Normal for age (prepubertal)	Normal – slightly increased estradiol
Premature adrenarche◇	Often girls 5-8 years old +/- slightly ↑ growth rate, + pubic hair, acne	Normal to slightly advanced bone age	Normal for age	Normal

* Best screening test for central precocious puberty. If high, suggests central. If low, suggests prepubertal or peripheral precocious puberty.

† Must differentiate from neonatal breast hyperplasia: Either sex can be affected. Subsides over weeks-months. Isolated finding and usually nonprogressive but 10% may advance to precocious puberty. Most resolve within 4 years.

◇ African American girls and small-for-gestational-age babies at risk. Up to 20% may develop polycystic ovary syndrome (PCOS) or hyperandrogenism later. Differentiate from congenital adrenal hyperplasia or adrenal tumors if abnormal exam or ↑17-OH progesterone (ACTH stimulation test or urine pregnanetriol).

PUBERTY CONTINUED

DIFFERENTIAL DIAGNOSIS of PRECOCIOUS PUBERTY

ISOSEXUAL		HETEROSEXUAL	
(development of secondary sexual characteristics consistent with patient's gender)		(development of secondary sexual characteristics consistent with opposite gender)	
CENTRAL	PERIPHERAL	GIRLS	BOYS
•Idiopathic	•Gonadal/ adrenal tumors*	•CAH	•Adolescent gynecomastia
•Hypothalamic hamartoma	•hCG or LH secreting tumors**	•Masculinizing tumors	•Klinefelter's syndrome
•Congenital CNS anomaly	•McCune-Albright	•Exogenous androgens	•Feminizing tumors
•CNS trauma	•CAH (↑DHEA-s)	•Idiopathic hirsutism	•Exogenous estrogens
•Neurofibromatosis	•Hypothyroidism	•Polycystic ovarian syndrome	•Marijuana use
•Prolonged CAH or sex steroid exposure	•Exogenous hormones		
•Russell-Silver syndrome	•Isolated premature thelarche or adrenarche		
	•Aromatase excess		

CNS: central nervous system; CAH: congenital adrenal hyperplasia; DHEA-s: dehydroepiandrosterone sulfate; hCG: human chorionic gonadotropin; LH: luteinizing hormone
*Adrenal/ovarian carcinoma or adenoma, granulosa cell tumor, theca cell tumor, Leydig cell tumor
**Choriocarcinoma, dysgerminoma, hepatoblastoma, chorioepithelioma, teratoma, gonadoblastoma

EVALUATION

▶ Thorough history, physical, neurologic, funduscopic and visual fields exam
▶ Assessment of height, weight, growth velocity, and Tanner staging
▶ Bone age x-rays (left hand/ wrist), dehydroepiandrosterone sulfate, 17-OH progesterone (if normal, congenital adrenal hyperplasia ruled out, if elevated, consider cosyntropin stimulation test), luteinizing hormone, follicle stimulating hormone, testosterone (♂), estradiol (♀), thyroid stimulating hormone, thyroxine
▶ Urine hCG if suspect hCG producing tumor
▶ Head CT or MRI (preferred) if true central precocious puberty (consider even if no neurologic signs, especially in boys)
▶ Pelvic/ abdominal ultrasound if gonadal or adrenal tumor is suspected; increased uterus length/ size suggests puberty
▶ Gonadotropin-releasing hormone agonist (GnRH, leuprolide) stimulation test to differentiate central from peripheral precocious puberty (if necessary)
▶ Adrenocorticotropic hormone (ACTH) stimulation test to identify adrenal cause

PUBERTY CONTINUED

TREATMENT

▶ Goal is to treat underlying cause (if identified), preserve adult height and ↓ psychosocial effects
▶ Gonadotropin-releasing hormone (GnRH) agonists are mainstay of therapy for idiopathic central precocious puberty.
▶ Medications such as ketoconazole, spironolactone, testolactone and tamoxifen may help limit effects of increased sex steroids, but formal evidence is lacking.

DELAYED PUBERTY

▶ Girls: Absence of secondary sex characteristics by 13 years old, or no menarche by age 16 (or within 5 years of onset of thelarche).
▶ Boys: Absence of secondary sexual characteristics by 14 years old.

DIFFERENTIAL DIAGNOSIS of DELAYED PUBERTY

Functional Hypogonadotropic Hypogonadism	Permanent Hypogonadotropic Hypogonadism	Hypergonadotropic Hypogonadism
Systemic illness	CNS tumors, infection, trauma	Klinefelter's syndrome (XXY)
Constitutional delay of growth and maturation*	CNS malformations	Turner & Noonan syndromes
Malnutrition/ eating disorders	Genetic syndromes (including CHARGE, Prader- Willi)	Gonadal trauma, torsion, infection (mumps)
Exercise (in excess)	Chemo/ radiation	Cryptorchidism
Endocrinopathies, including hypothyroidism	Kallmann syndrome (associated anosmia)	Androgen insensitivity
		5-α reductase deficiency

*More common in boys, usually with family history of "late bloomer".
CHARGE: Coloboma, heart defects, atresia of choanae, growth retardation, genitourinary & ear anomalies

EVALUATION

▶ Thorough history, family history, physical and neurologic examination
▶ Assessment of height, weight, and growth velocity
▶ Screening tests may include bone age x-rays (delayed), leuteinizing hormone (LH), follicle stimulating hormone (↑in hypergonadotropic), testosterone, estradiol, thyroid stimulating hormone (TSH), thyroxine (T4), CBC, ESR, comprehensive metabolic panel to evaluate liver and renal function, urinalysis, karyotype, celiac screen.

TREATMENT

▶ Testosterone or estrogen therapy may be indicated, especially to decrease the associated psychosocial stress of delayed puberty.
▶ Fertility can be induced with gonadotropin therapy in some patients with permanent hypogonadotropic hypogonadism.

Endocrinol Metab Clin North Am - 01-SEP-2005; 34(3): 617-41; Pediatrics 2002 Jan; 109(1): 61-7

ACUTE OTITIS MEDIA (AOM)

EPIDEMIOLOGY
▶ Risk factors: Bottle propping, smoke exposure, pacifier use, daycare, non-breastfed
▶ Decrease in AOM rates by 20% since routine use of PCV (*Prevnar*) vaccine
▶ Pathogens: ↓ vaccine serotypes of *Streptococcus pneumoniae*, ↑ non-vaccine serotypes of *S. Pneumo*, ↑non-typeable *Haemophilus influenzae* (H Flu), ↑ *Moraxella Catarrhalis*. Otitis-conjunctivitis syndrome: non-typeable *H. Flu*.

DIAGNOSIS OF ACUTE OTITIS MEDIA
▶ Clinical history alone is not well predictive of AOM.
▶ <u>AAP criteria</u>: *Acute onset* of signs and symptoms (otalgia, fussiness, crying, pain); presence of *middle ear fluid* [bulging or ↓ mobility of tympanic membrane (TM), air-fluid level, otorrhea]; *inflammation* of middle ear (inflamed TM, otalgia)

RECURRENT OTITIS MEDIA
▶ Recurrence within 7 days of completing antibiotics: More likely to be same pathogen; if 22-28 days after treatment 90% chance of being new pathogen.
▶ Non-typeable *H.Flu* is most likely pathogen to cause persistent/ recurrent AOM.
▶ Consider ENT referral if > 3 episodes/ 6 mo, > 4 episodes/ year, or hearing loss.

TREATMENT
▶ Pain control: acetaminophen, ibuprofen, topical drops
▶ Antibiotics ↓duration of symptoms, recurrence risk, and complications, especially in kids < 2 years. Should improve within 48-72 hours if on appropriate antibiotic.
▶ "Watchful waiting" may be considered in 1) kids > 2 years old with minimal symptoms or 2) kids > 6 mos old if diagnosis is uncertain (and non-severe illness) **and** close followup ensured. May consider prescribing antibiotics for parents to begin if symptoms do not improve (or worsen) during "watchful waiting" period.
▶ Symptoms will resolve in 75% of kids by 7 days regardless of treatment.

Antibiotic Options for Acute Otitis media

First Line	Amoxicillin 80-90 mg/kg/day divided bid
Penicillin (PCN) allergy (non-anaphylactic)	cefdinir (*Omnicef* = 14 mg/kg daily or divided bid), or cefpodoxime (10 mg/kg PO daily), or cefuroxime (30 mg/kg/day divided bid)
Penicillin Allergy (hives, anaphylaxis)	azithromycin standard dosing or consider 20 mg/kg/day x 3 days; or clarithromycin 15 mg/kg/day divided bid.
Refractory cases or initial treatment in severe cases	amoxicillin/ clavulanate 90/ 6.4 mg/kg/day divided bid, or cefdinir 14 mg/kg/day daily-bid or ceftriaxone 50 mg/kg IM (x 1-3 doses). Clindamycin + sulfonamide for PCN allergic
Treat for 10 days in most cases. 5-7 day treatment for kids > 6 years old with mild illness.	

COMPLICATIONS: Persistent middle ear fluid (recheck at 1-3 months after treatment), hearing loss, speech delay, balance problems, tinnitus, Bell's Palsy. Mastoiditis is rare, but requires immediate hospitalization and ENT consult.

Pediatric Clinics of North America 2005(52);3

OTITIS MEDIA WITH EFFUSION (OME)

Definition: Middle ear fluid without evidence of acute inflammation

Diagnosis: Physical examination, pneumatic otoscopy, tympanogram (81% sensitive and 74% specific in detecting OME)

Complications: Persistent OME may lead to problems with recurrent acute otitis media, hearing, behavior, vestibular function, gross motor coordination, sleep, tympanic membrane retraction pockets (posterosuperior), ossicular erosion, adhesive atelectasis of tympanic membrane, or cholesteatoma.

AAP Management Recommendations:

Identify kids at "high risk" for developmental problems (they should receive prompt speech, language and hearing evaluation, and possible ENT consultation).

HIGH RISK FOR DEVELOPMENTAL DELAY FROM COMPLICATIONS OF OME

●Developmental delay	●Visual impairment that is not correctable
●Speech delay	●Syndromes with craniofacial anomalies
●Down syndrome	●Syndromes with speech/ language difficulties
●Cleft palate	●Permanent hearing loss independent of OME

If child not "high risk" as defined above, consider the following management:

▶ **"Watchful waiting" for 3 months**

●Up to 90% of OME after acute otitis media will resolve at 3 months.
●55% of new-onset OME will *improve* at 3 months, but may recur.
●25% of new-onset OME (no acute otitis media) *resolves* at 3 months.

▶ **If OME persists beyond 3 months:**

●Continued "watchful waiting" may be appropriate, as 30% spontaneously resolve in < 12 months (in kids > 2 years old). Examine every 3-6 months.
●No long-term benefits of oral antibiotics (may try 1 course)

▶ **Risk factors for persistent OME** (not self resolving)

Onset in summer/ fall, hearing loss> 30 decibels, no history of adenoidectomy, prior tympanostomy tubes

▶ Antihistamines, decongestants, alternative medical therapies *not proven useful*.

HEARING EVALUATION

Evaluate hearing if OME > 3 months duration, or if learning difficulties, speech problems, or signs of decreased hearing.	
20-39 decibel hearing loss	Language evaluation; optimize listening-learning environment*, or tympanostomy tubes
> 40 decibel hearing loss	Language evaluation, tympanostomy tubes

* Optimizing listening-learning environment includes being close to and facing child when speaking, speaking slowly and clearly, turning off competing noise, and front -of -class seating.

OUTCOMES:

●After tympanostomy tubes, effusions ↓by 62% & hearing improves 8-12 decibels.
●20-50% will have relapse of OME after tubes out and may need replacement.
●Consider adenoidectomy if repeat tympanostomy tubes necessary

Adapted from AAP Clinical Practice Guideline: Otitis Media with Effusion, *Pediatrics* 2004 (113) 1412-1429.

OTITIS EXTERNA

▶ **Risk Factors:** Water exposure, trauma (foreign body, cotton swab), eczema, immunocompromised, use of hearing aids or earplugs.
▶ **Signs:** Otalgia, ↑ with manipulation of tragus or auricle.

TYPES OF OTITIS EXTERNA

Bacterial (swimmer's ear)	*Pseudomonas*; most common type (> 90% of acute otitis externa)
Fungal	*Aspergillus, candida*; ↑ in tropics or steroid drop use
Furunculosis	*S Aureus*; abscess in hair follicle; outer 1/3 of canal; may require draining abscess + topical antibiotics
Malignant	Advanced bacterial infection; requires systemic antibiotics & otolaryngology (ENT) consultation

TREATMENT

Prophylaxis or treatment of very mild cases	
Isopropyl alcohol (*Swim-Ear*)	4-5 drops (gtts) in ears after swimming
2% acetic acid (*VoSoL*)	or 3-5 gtts affected ear q 4-6 hours.

Topical antibiotics	
Ofloxacin (*Floxin Otic*) (> 6 months old)	5 gtts affected ear daily x 7 days

Topical antibiotics + steroids*	
Polymyxin/ neomycin/ HC (*Cortisporin Otic*)	3 gtts affected ear tid-qid x 5-10 d
Ciprofloxacin (*Cipro HC Otic*)	3 gtts affected ear bid x 7 days
Ciprofloxacin + dexamethasone (*CiproDex*)	4 gtts affected ear bid x 7 days

Topical antifungals	
Tolnaftate (*Tinactin*) or clotrimazole (*Lotrimin*) solution	Apply tid- qid x 5-10 days

Systemic antibiotics (malignant OE): Include anti-pseudomonal coverage

*Do not use if tympanostomy (PE) tubes or known/ suspected TM perforation.
HC= hydrocortisone   *Pediatr Clin North Am* 2006; 53(2): 195-214

CERUMEN REMOVAL

▶ Curette and lavage are generally safest and best options. If there is any doubt about integrity of TM (perforation, PE tubes), avoid using cerumenolytic agents.

CERUMENOLYTIC AGENTS (none FDA approved for use in children)

Docusate (*Colace liquid*)	1 mL in ear canal / let sit for 15 min.
Triethanolamine (*Cerumenex*)	Fill canal, let sit x 15 minutes, irrigate
Carbamide peroxide (*Debrox*)	5-10 gtts affected ear bid x 4 days

TYMPANIC MEMBRANE PERFORATION

Usually heal in 2-3 weeks spontaneously. Do not get wet. May use topical antibiotic if draining. Refer to ENT urgently if large perforation, vertigo, facial nerve paralysis, hearing loss, flaps of TM in toward middle ear (risk cholesteatoma) or if not healed spontaneously in 3 weeks.

Adapted from: Textbook of Pediatric Emergency Medicine, Ludwig & Fleisher, 4th ed, pp 1410

HEARING LOSS/ AUDIOLOGY

▶ 1-6/ 1000 newborns have significant congenital hearing loss. Early identification/ intervention (in first 6 months of life) may ↓ risk of poor outcome. Older kids should have regular screening; even unilateral/ mild hearing loss may be associated with social, emotional, and academic problems.

RISK FACTORS FOR HEARING LOSS

< 1 month old	Family history (50% genetic)[3], congenital toxoplasmosis, rubella, cytomegalovirus, herpes simplex virus, syphilis, craniofacial/ ear anomalies, bacterial meningitis, severe hyperbilirubinemia, low apgar (0-3, 0-6), birth weight < 1500 g, respiratory distress, birth asphyxia, mechanical ventilation > 10 days, ototoxic medications > 5 days (loop diuretics, gentamicin); syndromes: Down, Waardenburg, Treacher-Collins, Crouzon, fetal alcohol, Alport
1 month – 2 years old	Any of the above, delayed speech/ language development, parental concern about hearing, recurrent/ persistent ear effusion (>3 months), temporal bone fracture (trauma), measles, mumps, neurodegenerative disorders (mucopolysaccharidoses), demyelinating diseases (Friedrich ataxia, Charcot-Marie-Tooth)

PHYSICAL EXAMINATION: Heterochromia of irises (Waardenburg syndrome), auricular/ ear canal malformation, preauricular dimples/ skin tags, cleft lip/palate, facial asymmetry/ hypoplasia, microcephaly, tympanic membrane anomalies

OBJECTIVE HEARING ASSESSMENT

Test Name	Age / Time	Details
Auditory brainstem response (ABR)*	Any age; (newborn) 15 minutes	Measures nerve/ brainstem activity in response to frequencies > 1000Hz; electrodes on head. Ear specific results. Pass/ Fail score. Best results if child is sleeping.
Evoked otoacoustic emissions	Any age; 10 minutes	Otoacoustic emissions (OAE) are made in response to clicks; probes in ears; fails test if no OAE for threshold > 30 dB
Conditioned oriented responses (COR)	Minimum 9-12 months; > 30 min	Child learns to associate sound with reinforcement & their behavior tells you what they hear/ understand. Also: Visual reinforced audiometry (*VRA*)
Play audiometry	2-4 years; >30 min.	Teach to respond to sound with play activity (drop block in box when you hear sound)
Conventional audiometry	> 4 years; 10 min	Air: Raise hand in response to sound, tested 500-4000 Hz. 50% with normal hearing hear 0 dB. Normal speech at 45 dB. BONE: Vibrators on mastoid process, tests inner ear sensitivity.

*OAE and ABR do not assess cortical processing of sound.

AUDIOLOGY CONTINUED

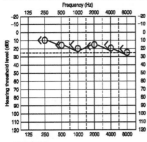

NORMAL AUDIOGRAM

-10-25 dB: normal hearing
26-40 dB: mild hearing loss
41-55 dB: mod hearing loss
56-70 dB: mod- severe loss
71-90 dB: severe hearing loss
>90 dB: profound hearing loss

Audiogram Key

Test	Right ear
Air	O
Bone mastoid unmasked	<

From The Merck Manual of Diagnosis and Therapy, Edition 18, p. 786, edited by Mark H. Beers. Copyright 2006 by Merck & Co., Inc., Whitehouse Station , NJ . Available at: www.merck.com. Accessed 4/28/07.

Sensorineural hearing loss: ↓ air and bone conduction
Conductive hearing loss: ↓ air conduction, normal bone conduction
Mixed hearing loss: ↓ air and bone conduction, but may be different degrees

INTERVENTIONS:

► Repeat any failed screen (after treatment if indicated for acute otitis media).
► If child fails hearing screen twice, refer to audiologist comprehensive evaluation.
► Chronic/recurrent otitis media with effusion (OME) + failed screen: Refer to ENT.
► Sensorineural hearing loss: Refer to audiology and ENT for possible hearing aid.
► Appropriate speech/ language therapy and other behavioral interventions as needed.

TYMPANOGRAMS: Can help detect presence of middle ear effusion or retracted tympanic membrane (TM).

Type A: Normal (central peak)
Type B: Flat (may be associated with large ear canal volumes, middle ear fluid, PE tubes or perforation)
Type C: Negative, left-shifted peak (may be associated with retracted TM's)

1. *Pediatrics* 2003.111 (2): 436-440 2. www.audiologyawareness.com/hhelp/audiogrm.htm 3. Canalis, R.F. & Lambert, P.R. (2000). The Ear: Comprehensive Otology. Philadelphia : Lippincott, Williams, Wilkins. (www.asha.org). See www.audiologyawareness.com or www.asha.org

SINUSITIS

SINUS DEVELOPMENT

Maxillary/ ethmoid sinuses:	Present at birth
Sphenoid sinuses:	Develop between 5-7 years of age
Frontal sinuses:	By age 18 years. 20% of adults have only 1

RISK FACTORS: Upper respiratory infection (URI), allergic rhinitis, dry air, craniofacial anomalies, deviated nasal septum, nasal foreign body, polyp (possible cystic fibrosis), large adenoids, gastroesophageal reflux disease, immune dysfunction (IgA deficiency, ciliary dyskinesia), hypersensitivity to airborne molds

SYMPTOMS: Nasal congestion, cough, headache & sinus pressure (in 33%), nasal obstruction, foul breath, fever, periorbital swelling, URI that does not improve after 10-14 days (~10% of URI complicated by sinusitis), fever >48 hrs into URI -type illness, cough worse at night; may see acute fever, facial/ sinus pain

CLASSIFICATION

Acute	< 30 days of symptoms
Subacute	Symptoms 30-90 days
Recurrent	3 episodes of acute bacterial sinusitis in 6 months or 4 episodes/12 months (10 days symptom free between episodes)
Chronic	> 90 days of continuous symptoms

ETIOLOGY: S pneumoniae (30-60%), H influenza (20-30%) M catarrhalis (12-30%)

WORKUP

▶ Sinus X-rays: Nonspecific and should not be used in kids < 6 years (88% positive if prolonged symptoms as above) and used sparingly in kids > 6 years (70% +)
▶ X-rays best initial study if necessary. 99% sensitive and 46% specific if one of the following: air–fluid levels, complete opacification, or mucosal thickening >4 mm.
▶ Consider computed tomography for recurrent, refractory, or complicated sinusitis.
▶ Skin test to environmental allergens (~ 50% + if chronic sinusitis) or IgE levels
▶ Other workup as appropriate if underlying problem suspected.

TREATMENT

▶ Amoxicillin 45 mg/ kg/ day if no daycare, no recent antibiotics, and > 2 years old.
▶ Amoxicillin 90 mg/ kg/ day + clavulanic acid if < 2 years old, daycare, recent antibiotics; second line agents: cefprozil, cefuroxime, azithromycin.
▶ Duration of treatment not well studied. AAP guidelines suggest treating for 7 days past resolution of symptoms (10-21 days).
▶ Consider nasal saline; no proven benefit of decongestants, nasal steroids, mucolytics.
▶ Surgery in complicated cases (adenoidectomy may improve 70-80% of cases)

COMPLICATIONS: Preseptal or orbital cellulitis; cavernous sinus thrombosis; subperiosteal abscess at frontal bone; subdural, epidural or brain abscess

Zacharisen M, Immunol Allergy Clin North Am, 2005; 25(2): 313-32

NASAL TRAUMA

▶ In child with nasal trauma, rule out associated injury to cervical spine, central nervous system, and eyes.
▶ Deformity usually indicates nasal fracture, but may be best evaluated by ENT in 2-4 days when ↓ swelling. May be reduced in < 1 week. X-rays unreliable.
▶ Consider antibiotics if suspect nose fracture: may communicate with nasal cavity.
▶ Red flags: Septal hematoma (drain to prevent complications such as saddle nose deformity), cerebral spinal fluid (CSF) rhinorrhea, suspected sinus trauma (crepitance, + x-rays), other associated injury.

EPISTAXIS

CAUSES

Nose picking, upper respiratory infection, allergies, dry environment. Also, trauma, foreign body, intranasal drug use, cancers (leukemia), chemotherapy, liver failure, idiopathic thrombocytopenia purpura, coagulopathies (hemophilia, von Willebrand's disease, Osler-Weber-Rendu, drugs)

WORKUP: (Prolonged, recurrent, red flags)

•Complete blood count
•Prothrombin time (PT), partial thromboplastin time (PTT), von Willebrand's panel, liver function studies as indicated by history and physical examination.

MANAGEMENT:

•Pressure (pinching nose) and/ or cotton roll under upper lip
• Insert vasoconstrictor- (Neo-Synephrine or Afrin) soaked cotton if continues.
• Consult ENT for cautery, Gelfoam/ Surgicel or posterior pack if persists.

Pediatr Clin North Am - 01-APR-2006; 53(2): 195-214

CLEFT LIP & PALATE

•May involve lip, alveolar tissue, and/or palate in varying degrees of severity.
•Early in-utero defect: Lip fuses by 5 weeks, palate by 8-9 weeks gestation
•Incidence: Unilateral (left > right) > bilateral > midline (rare)
•Racial incidence disparity: Asian > Hispanic = Caucasian > African American

Risk of recurrence in future children	
Unaffected parents	4%
1 affected parent	4%
1 parent & 1 child affected	10-15%

Risk of concurrent syndrome	
Isolated cleft lip	Low
Cleft lip & palate	Med
Isolated cleft palate	High

•Refer immediately to nearest interdisciplinary team & geneticist to guide care.
•Feeding difficulties: Soft nipple with large opening or squeezable bottles help.
•Staged Repair: Lip @ 3 months, palate <12-18 months (+/- tympanotomy tubes)
•Complications: Hearing loss, otitis media, speech difficulties, dental anomalies common.

PHARYNGITIS

ETIOLOGY

▶ Usually viral [influenza, parainfluenza, adenovirus, rhinovirus, Epstein-Barr virus (EBV), herpes, coxsackie], especially if accompanied by coryza, conjunctivitis, low-grade fever, diarrhea or vomiting.

▶ 15-30% of pharyngitis in children, and 10% in adults, caused by Group A Strep. Up to 30% of kids with EBV may also have strep infection (if both, treat strep with an antibiotic other than amoxicillin).

▶ Other bacterial causes: Group C or G beta-hemolytic strep (can cause epidemic food-borne pharyngitis; usually in eggs, milk), *Corynebacterium*, *N. gonorrhoeae*

PRESENTATION
Clinical Findings of various types of pharyngitis

Strep A, C, G	Fever, sore throat, headache, enlarged, tender anterior cervical nodes, beefy red swollen uvula, tonsillar/ pharyngeal erythema +/- exudate, bad breath, scarlatiniform rash*, petechiae on palate, "strawberry tongue" Usually no congestion/ cough More common in patients < 15 years old Pharyngeal exudate and history of strep exposure are most predictive of strep
Adenovirus	May be associated with conjunctivitis ("pharyngoconjunctival fever"), nasal congestion; otherwise may look similar to strep
Coxsackie A & B/ Echoviruses	Papulovesicles on erythematous base in oropharynx Coxsackie A16 causes "hand-foot-mouth disease", with lesions on palms & soles Exudate and tender adenopathy uncommon
Epstein-Barr Virus (EBV)/ Mononucleosis	Can look identical to Strep Posterior adenopathy common May also have diffuse lymphadenopathy and hepatomegaly (8%) or splenomegaly (17%) If treated with amoxicillin, 90% develop maculopapular rash
Diphtheria	Grayish membrane in pharynx.
Gonorrhea	Sexually active adolescents; green exudates; may also have dysuria, arthritis Throat culture on Thayer-Martin media if suspected

* Scarlatiniform rash: Erythematous and sandpaper-like; usually starts near neck and spreads to trunk/ legs/ arms. Desquamates after 3-4 days.

STREP CARRIERS

▶ Up to 20% of kids might be Strep carriers. Very low risk of infecting contacts or developing complications. No evidence of immune response.

PHARYNGITIS CONTINUED

STUDIES: Laboratory aids used in the diagnosis of pharyngitis

Test	Sensitivity	Specificity	Comments
Strep pharyngitis			
Throat culture	90-95%	99%	Final read at 48 hours. Group C & G grow in anaerobic incubation.
Rapid strep antigen	80-90%[1]	95%[1]	Will miss C & G Strep; consider culture if negative.
Infectious Mononucleosis [Epstein-Barr Virus (EBV)]			
CBC with differential	61% (EBV)	95% (EBV)	Aids in diagnosis of EBV; >50% lymphocytes (> 10% atypical)
Heterophile antibodies "Monospot test"	86%	91%	Lower sensitivity in kids < 12 years old and first 2 weeks of illness
EBV viral capsid antigen antibodies	97%	94%	Consider if clinical picture highly suggestive but heterophile antibodies negative (IgM = acute infection, IgG only = immunity)
EBV nuclear antigen antibodies	97%	94%	Usually not positive until 6 weeks after illness; helps determine if recent or past illness.

COMPLICATIONS:

▶ *Strep:* Retropharyngeal abscess (nuchal rigidity, toxic appearance), peritonsillar abscess (< 1% of those treated with antibiotics; "hot potato voice", uvula deviation, drooling, fluctuant mass), otitis media, sinusitis, post -strep glomerulonephritis, acute rheumatic fever [(ARF) < 1/100,000 in United States], lymphadenitis, meningitis, bacteremia, endocarditis.

▶ *Mononucleosis:* Splenic rupture in 0.1 % of patients. Other rare complications include nephritis, neurologic problems, cardiac conduction problems, hemolytic anemia, thrombocytopenia.

TREATMENT:

▶ General: Pain control, antipyretics, and maintain hydration.

▶ *Strep pharyngitis:* May delay treatment for 9 days after onset of symptoms and still prevent ARF. Treatment may ↓illness by 1 day. Goal is to avoid complications. Only IM penicillin shown to prevent ARF in controlled studies, but as many other antibiotics eradicate Strep, it is assumed that they also work to prevent ARF. Antibiotics do not change risk of post-strep glomerulonephritis. May return to work/ school after afebrile and at least 24 hours of antibiotics.

▶ *Mononucleosis:* Avoid contact sports for at least 4 weeks *and* asymptomatic. No antivirals necessary. Corticosteroids rarely indicated for severe pharyngeal edema.

▶ Treatment for Group C and G Strep is controversial, but if patient is symptomatic, treatment is generally recommended.

PHARYNGITIS CONTINUED

Treatment options for Group A Streptococcal pharyngitis

Antibiotic (dosage forms)	Dose	Notes
Penicillin V (125 mg/5 mL or 250 mg/5mL solution; 250 mg or 500 mg tabs)	25-50 mg/kg/day divided qid x 10 days Adult dose: 500 mg PO bid or tid x 10 days	May use amoxicillin* 50 mg/kg/day divided tid x 10 days if taste preferred.
Penicillin G Benzathine (IM)* (600,000 units/ mL)	25,000-50,000 units/ kg IM (max 1.2 million units) single dose. Adults: 1.2 million units IM	Convenient, single dose treatment. Painful.
Erythromycin* (200 mg/5 mL, 400 mg/5 mL, 200 mg chewable tab or 400 mg tabs)	40 mg/kg/day divided qid x 10 days (max 1g/day) Adults: 400-800 mg PO q 6-12 hr x 10 days	For penicillin allergic. Beware multiple drug interactions. 10 days of treatment.
Cephalexin (125 mg/5 mL, 250 mg/5 mL, 250 mg or 500 mg tablet)	50 mg/kg/day divided qid x 10 days Adults: 250-500 mg PO q 6 hr x 10 days	May use in relapse, recurrent infection, or intolerance to penicillin.
Clindamycin (75 mg/5 mL, 75 mg, 150 mg or 300 mg capsules)	20-30 mg/kg/day divided tid x 10 days	Consider if penicillin allergic *and* unable to tolerate erythromycin or cephalexin. Small risk of pseudomembranous colitis.
Azithromycin (100 mg/5 mL, 200 mg/5 mL, 250 mg or 600 mg tablet)	12 mg/kg/day single daily dose (max 500 mg PO daily)	Treat for 5 days. Second line therapy.
Cefdinir (125 mg/5 mL, 250 mg/5 mL, 300 mg capsules)	14 mg/kg/day once daily, max 600 mg/day	10 day course

* Considered first-line and preferred therapies.

1. Gerber MA - *Pediatr Clin North Am* - 01-JUN-2005; 52(3): 729-47;
2. Ebell MH - *Am Fam Physician* - 1-OCT-2004; 70(7): 1279-87;
3. Vincent MT - *Am Fam Physician* - 15-MAR-2004; 69(6): 1465-70

NECK MASS		
CONGENITAL	Often present at birth, smooth, non-tender, cystic, soft, at risk for superinfection. Ultrasound/CT/MRI to confirm diagnosis.	
Thyroglossal duct cyst	Midline, inferior to hyoid, moves up with swallowing or tongue protrusion	Surgical excision including tract to tongue
Branchial cleft cyst	Lateral (anterior to middle 1/3 of sternocleidomastoid), occasional mucoid drainage	Treatment: Surgical excision
Cystic hygroma (lymphangioma)	75% posterior triangle of neck, 20% axillary, progressive growth	Poor outcome from surgery & sclerotherapy
Hemangioma	Gradual growth from birth, any location, spontaneously involute	Therapy only if causes vision, airway problems
Dermoid cyst	Subcutaneous, nodular, non-tender	Excision

INFECTIOUS	
INFECTIOUS	Reactive lymphadenopathy present in ~50% all healthy children. Often tender; recent pharyngitis, skin, ear, dental infection.
Viral	Epstein-Barr virus (EBV), adenovirus, roseola, cytomegalovirus (CMV), upper respiratory infection, enterovirus
Bacterial	Lymphadenitis: *Staph aureus* & Group A Streptococcus (75%): Unilateral, tender, warm, red. Treatment: Dicloxacillin, cephalexin, amoxicillin/ clavulanate
	Cat Scratch disease (Bartonella): Subacute, non-tender, occasional hepatosplenomegaly. No treatment generally needed. Can use rifampin or trimethoprim/sulfamethoxazole.
	Deep neck infection: Parapharyngeal, retropharyngeal, peritonsillar abscess. Requires surgical drainage +/- antibiotics.
	Sialadenitis: Rare in children, polymicrobial, red, swollen, tender submandibular mass. Treatment: Hydration, *Augmentin*.
Mycobacterial	Tuberculosis: Multiple, bilateral, non-tender.
	Atypical: Non-tender, firm, unilateral, child < 5 years old. No response to antibiotics. No treatment generally necessary. Consider excision.
Other	Toxoplasmosis, human immunodeficiency virus (HIV), actinomycosis, coccidiomycosis

ONCOLOGIC		
ONCOLOGIC	Slow growing, unilateral, firm, deep, non-tender, and/or fixed. Consider biopsy if supraclavicular, lower 1/3 of neck, gradual ↑size, no regression by 6-8 weeks, weight loss.	
Benign	Lipoma, neurofibroma, keloids	Excision or watchful waiting
Malignant	Hodgkin's (or non-Hodgkin's) lymphoma, neuroblastoma	Concern if supraclavicular or lower 2/3 neck

OTHER	Kawasaki disease: Unilateral, >1.5 cm, associated fever.
Benign adenopathy: no systemic symptoms, < 1 cm, mobile, "rubbery", no growth	

ACUTE ABDOMINAL PAIN

| Obstruction: Emesis (bilious) Peritonitis: Guarding, rebound, percussion or point tenderness See below table. | **Trauma?** No ⟶ Yes ⟶ | Emergent evaluation for hematoma, hemorrhage, perforated viscus, and/or contusion |

DIFFERENTIAL DIAGNOSIS*

• Intussusception	• Appendicitis	• Gastroenteritis
• Cystic fibrosis	• Bowel infarction	• Hepatitis
• Volvulus	• Cholecystitis	• Henoch-Schönlein purpura
• Incarcerated hernia	• Ectopic pregnancy	• Urinary tract infection
• Pelvic inflammatory disease	• Volvulus	• Pneumonia
		• Ruptured ovarian cyst

*Each specific illness may present with a variety of clinical signs or symptoms.

DIFFERENTIAL DIAGNOSIS BY LOCATION OF PAIN

Right upper quadrant	• Hepatitis, cholecystitis, acute cholangitis, pyelonephritis, gastritis, pneumonia, nephrolithiasis, pleural effusion, pericarditis, pancreatitis, gastroenteritis, constipation
Right lower quadrant	• Appendicitis, gastroenteritis, constipation, ovarian pain, ectopic pregnancy, inflammatory bowel disease, testicular torsion, hernia
Epigastric	• Gastritis, gastroenteritis, gastroesophageal reflux, peptic ulcer disease, pancreatitis, pneumonia, pericarditis, constipation
Peri-umbilical	• Gastroenteritis, constipation, early appendicitis, urinary tract infection, obstruction, fever, irritable bowel syndrome, lead/iron toxicity, inflammatory bowel disease, mesenteric adenitis
Left upper quadrant	• Constipation, pancreatitis, pyelonephritis, pneumonia, pericarditis, nephrolithiasis, pleural effusion, splenomegaly, hydronephrosis, gastroenteritis
Left lower quadrant	• Constipation, gastroenteritis, inflammatory bowel disease, ovarian pain, ectopic pregnancy, hernia, testicular torsion
Suprapubic	• Cystitis, constipation, pelvic inflammatory disease, urinary tract infection, gastroenteritis

ACUTE APPENDICITIS: If diagnosis unclear by exam and labs, consider imaging:

CRP & WBC	↑values suggestive, but not diagnostic, of appendicitis	
Ultrasound	PPV=91%	NPV=88%	If negative, consider CT
CT with contrast	PPV=92%	NPV=98%	IV, PO, and/or rectal contrast Radiology. 2002 Jun;223(3):633-8

CT=computed tomography, NPV=negative predictive value, PPV=positive predictive value

CHRONIC ABDOMINAL PAIN

•**Characteristics**: Episodic (≥3 episodes in 3 months), self-limited (<1-3 hours), poorly localized pain, frequently peri-umbilical and unrelated to meals or activity. May have nausea and/or vomiting. Often interferes with activities and school attendance. Complex interaction with familial psychosocial issues.

Functional:	No identifiable cause. Possible syndromes: Abdominal migraine, irritable bowel syndrome, functional dyspepsia, functional abdominal pain.
Organic:	Presumed anatomic, infectious, inflammatory or metabolic cause

Approach to chronic abdominal pain
Thorough history & physical exam focusing on "Red Flags"

Historical "Red Flags"	*Physical Exam "Red Flags"*
•Bilious or intractable emesis	•Organomegaly
•Epigastric or right-sided pain	•Abdominal mass
•Loss of appetite or recurrent fever	•Localized abdominal tenderness
•Patient ≤ 4 years old	•Decreased height velocity
•Night awakening	•Arthritis (swelling, redness, warmth)
•Radiation to back	•Peri-rectal fistula or skin tag
•Family history of inflammatory bowel disease	•Frank or occult blood in stool
•Dysuria	•Rash

Pediatrics, Vol. 115 No. 3 March 2005, pp. 812-815

Consider CBC, ESR, urinalysis, stool occult blood in all patients

+ Screening labs and/or "red flags"

•Further diagnostic studies (see table below)
•Consider gastroenterologist consult

Negative screening labs and no "red flags": <2% will have organic cause. Chronic pain syndromes: Abdominal migraine, irritable bowel syndrome, functional dyspepsia, functional pain

Upper GI series +/- endoscopy	•Consider in patients with epigastric pain suspicious for peptic ulcer disease.
Blood tests	•Serum albumin, liver & renal function. Gastroenterologist may recommend inflammatory bowel disease panel.
Ultrasound	•Consider if patient has abdominal mass, dysuria, colicky pain, flank pain
Stool studies	•Ova & parasite examination if diarrhea prominent

CBC=complete blood count, ESR=erythrocyte sedimentation rate, IBD=inflammatory bowel disease

GASTROINTESTINAL (GI) BLEEDING

Age	Upper GI Bleed (UGI)	Lower GI Bleed (LGI)
< 1 mo old	•Ingested maternal blood, esophagitis, bleeding disorder, gastric ulcer	•Cow's milk/ soy protein intolerance, anal fissure, ingested maternal blood, infection, bowel ischemia (necrotizing enterocolitis, volvulus), upper GI bleed
1 month-2 years old	•Gastritis, esophagitis, ulcer	•Fissure, cow's milk/ soy protein intolerance, infection, ischemia, intussusception, polyps, Meckel's
2-5 years old	•Gastritis, esophagitis, ulcer, varices, bleeding diathesis	•Red food/medication ingestion (cefdinir), fissure, infection, foreign body, polyp, Meckel's, intussusception, bowel ischemia, inflammatory bowel disease
> 5 years old	•Peptic ulcer, gastritis, esophagitis	•Infection (bacterial, viral, parasitic), inflammatory bowel disease, Meckel's, red food/medication ingestion, polyp, hemorrhoid, fissure

GI: Gastrointestinal, IBD: Inflammatory Bowel Disease, NEC: Necrotizing enterocolitis,

INTUSSUSCEPTION

Pathology	Epidemiology
•Telescoping of bowel •Proximal→distal segment •Engorged veins, edema and ischemia	•95% ileocolic (at ileocolic junction) •5% ileoileal: Associated with Meckel diverticulum and Henoch-Schönlein purpura •80% patients <2 years old, ♂:♀ = 2:1

Clinical signs (<10% patients present with ≥3 of the below)
•Paroxysms of severe pain, interspersed with symptom free periods
•Vomiting (occasionally bilious)
•Bloody stool: ~70% patients + for occult or gross blood. "Currant jelly stool" is a late sign.
•Right upper quadrant mass

Diagnosis	Treatment Options	
•Air or barium enema •Ultrasound sensitive (especially for ileoileal) •X-rays low yield	**Air or hydrostatic enema** % Success by duration illness <48 hours: 70-90% >48 hours: <50%	**Surgical reduction** •1st line for patients with perforation, shock, peritonitis, or ileoileal intussusception

Post-reduction management: Hospitalize for observation given recurrence risk
•5-8% recurrence risk post-enema (treat as 1st episode)
•2-5% recurrence risk post-surgical reduction
•Low morbidity to recurrence at home

CONSTIPATION

NORMAL STOOL FREQUENCY

Age	Range (stools/ week)	Mean (stools/day)	
0-3 months breastfed	5-40	3	*Some normal children have 1 stool every 4-5 days; if it is soft & does not cause distress, most likely not concerning.
0-3 months, formula	5-25	2	
6-12 months	5-28	1.8	
1-3 years	4-21	1.4	
> 3 years	3-14	1	

HISTORICAL CLUES TO ASK ABOUT

Weight loss/ anorexia	Vomiting	Encopresis	Delayed meconium
Onset in infancy	Rectal pain/ bleeding		Withholding behavior
Family history of hypothyroidism, Hirschsprung's, cystic fibrosis, celiac disease			

DIFFERENTIAL DIAGNOSIS

Nonorganic*	Low fiber diet, dehydration, psychosocial, withholding
Anatomic causes	Imperforate anus, anal stenosis, displaced anus, mass
Metabolic Causes	Hypothyroidism, hypercalcemia, hypokalemia, diabetes
Spinal Cord anomalies	Tethered cord, spinal trauma or mass
Food intolerance	Gluten enteropathy, cow's milk protein intolerance
Other disorders	Cystic fibrosis, Hirschsprung's, NF, CP, prune belly, gastroschisis, Down syndrome, connective tissue disease
Drugs	Opiates, phenobarbital, antacids, antidepressants, iron
Infection/ toxic	Botulism, lead/ heavy metal ingestion, vitamin D

*most common cause, even in infants; CP: Cerebral palsy; NF: Neurofibromatosis

PHYSICAL EXAM RED FLAGS

Abdomen distended	Patulous anus	Displaced anus	Failure to thrive
Absent anal wink	Explosive stool	Occult blood	Anal skin tags
Back: midline hair tuft, dimple, pigment changes, no lumbar-sacral curve		Neuro: muscle atrophy/ flat buttocks, ↓ strength/ tone lower extremities, altered deep tendon reflexes	

WORKUP

► Abdominal X-rays if unable to do rectal exam, or history consistent with constipation but exam normal.
► Barium or air contrast enema, rectal manometry, and/or rectal biopsy if suspect Hirschsprung's disease
► Consider thyroid stimulating hormone (TSH), thyroxine (T4), calcium, celiac antibodies (see pp. 84), lead, colonic transport study, sweat chloride, and/or psychological evaluation if clinically indicated. In refractory cases, consider MRI of lumbosacral spine (tethered cord, sacral agenesis, tumor).

TREATMENT

► Education, disimpaction and maintenance
► Disimpaction may be done as in- or outpatient depending on severity/ situation.
► If encopresis is present, see section on encopresis pp. 37

CONSTIPATION CONTINUED

DISIMPACTION

Age group	Suggestions
Infants	• Enemas not recommended • Glycerin suppositories may be used occasionally
Older kids/ adolescents	ORAL: Polyethylene glycol 3350 (MiraLax), mineral oil† (> 5 yr) RECTAL: No consensus about digital disimpaction; mineral oil, saline, phosphate soda enemas; bisacodyl suppository (Avoid tap water, soap suds, magnesium enemas)

MAINTENANCE

Infants	Dietary Changes: 2-4 oz/ day of apple, prune, pear juice	Medications: Lactulose, corn syrup, sorbitol, barley malt extract (AVOID mineral oil or stimulant laxatives)	
Older Kids/ Adolescents	Dietary Changes: High Fiber diet (age in years)+ 5= goal grams of fiber /day; stay hydrated; add high sorbitol juices	Behavioral Changes: Unhurried time on toilet after meals. Do not withhold. Do not scold.	Medications: Mineral oil, mag hydroxide, lactulose, sorbitol, polyethylene glycol 3350 (MiraLax)

MEDICATIONS COMMONLY USED IN THE TREATMENT OF CONSTIPATION

MEDICATION	DOSE	NOTES
Phosphate Enemas (Fleet)	2-11 years: 2.25 oz Pediatric enema PR >12 years: 4.5 oz enema PR.	Avoid in kids < 2 years old, history of kidney or cardiac disease
Mineral Oil Enema	2-11 years old: 30-60 mL >12 years: 60-150 mL PR	Avoid if ostomy or appendicitis
Polyethylene Glycol solution (GoLYTELY)	25 mL/ kg/ hr (max 1000 mL/ hr) by nasogastric until clear	Usually inpatient (for disimpaction)
Mineral Oil†	1-3 mL/kg/d divided qd-tid	Kids > 4 years old only
Lactulose (10g/ 15 mL syrup)	infants: 2.5-10 mL PO daily older children: 1-3 mL/ kg/ day divided bid	Avoid in galactosemia and diabetes mellitus
Magnesium Citrate 1.745 g/30 ml	> 2 years: 2-4 mL/kg/day PO div qd-bid; max 150 ml/day	Avoid in renal dysfunction, acute abdomen
Malt Soup Extract (Barley Malt Extract)	infants: 1-2 teaspoons in 2-4 oz formula or water qd-bid	
Polyethylene Glycol 3350 (MiraLax)	½- 1 tablespoon full in 8 oz water daily	As with all medications, avoid prolonged use.

†Risk of lipoid pneumonia if aspirated. Use only in neurologically normal children >4 years old.

ACUTE DIARRHEA

Diarrhea-related dehydration = 10% of hospital admissions in children < 5 yrs old.
Differential diagnosis: Viral or bacterial enteritis, parasitic infections, transient lactase deficiency, overfeeding, starvation diarrhea, toddler's diarrhea
Assessment: Rule out emergent conditions, assess hydration status
Management: Prevention, sanitation, handwashing, vaccines, isolation, rehydration

VIRAL CAUSES OF ACUTE DIARRHEA

Virus	Symptoms	Illness duration/ Viral shedding	Commonly affected / Other
Rotavirus	•Fever, emesis, diarrhea •10-20 green, foul smelling stools/ day	•3-8 days of symptoms •May shed virus for 21 days	•Children 4-24 months •Infected adult contacts may be asymptomatic •Stool antigen test and vaccine available
Caliciviruses (norovirus)	•Vomiting, diarrhea and cramps •Occasional low-grade fever	•Symptoms last up to 3 days	•Most common cause of viral diarrhea outbreaks (schools, cruise ships, institutions)
Astroviruses	•Diarrhea, vomiting, fever •Occasionally asymptomatic	•4-5 days •May shed virus for days-weeks	•Children < 4 years old •Usually in winter months
Enteric adenoviruses	•Diarrhea, vomiting, low-grade fever	•Days-weeks •Contagious during acute illness	•Children < 4 years old •High fever uncommon (unlike non-enteric adenoviruses)

OTHER NON-BACTERIAL CAUSES OF ACUTE DIARRHEA

Antibiotic associated	•2 days-2 months after antibiotics •Common offending antibiotics: Penicillins +/- clavulanate, cephalosporins, clindamycin	•Usually self-limited and mild •Probiotics* may ↓incidence[1]; not routinely recommended •Cefdinir may make stools dark red, (though guaiac negative)
Post-infectious	•Brush border denudation may lead to transient disaccharidase deficiency and malabsorptive state	

*S. boulardii, Lactobacillus GG, and combination of B. lactis and S. thermophilus.
1. Journal of Pediatrics 149 (3) 9/06

BACTERIAL CAUSES OF ACUTE DIARRHEA

Pathogen	Transmission	Presentation	Treatment	Other
Campylobacter	•Poultry, dogs, cats, contaminated water, fecal material; person to person less common	•Variable; +/- fever, cramps in 66%, bloody stool in >50% •80% of cases last < 1 week •Incubation 1-7 days	Most do not require abx Erytho or azithromycin x 5-7 days may ↓ duration of symptoms	•Eradication after 2-3 days of antibiotics •↑ risk Guillain-Barré syndrome
Escherichia coli	•Person-person, contaminated water & food, unpasteurized milk •0157:H7: Ground beef, petting zoos, apple cider, raw fruits and vegetables, contaminated water •Incubation: 1-8 days. •Excreted up to 2 weeks	•Enterohemorrhagic E Coli: Fever (33%), severe abdominal pain, bloody stools •0157:H7: 8% of patients develop hemolytic uremic syndrome (HUS) •Other types: "Traveler's diarrhea" days→weeks of watery diarrhea and cramps, self-limited	•Treat severe disease with TMP-SMX, azithromycin or ciprofloxacin for 3 days •Antibiotics for 0157:H7: No proven benefit. Meta-analysis did not confirm ↑ risk of HUS if used.	•HUS: Onset <2 wks after illness: Renal failure, hemolytic anemia, ↓platelet. •If labs normal 3 days after resolution, low risk of HUS. •↑risk diabetes mellitus after HUS.
Shigella	•Person-person, contaminated water	•Tenesmus, high-fever (40°C), watery→bloody diarrhea	•Ampicillin, TMP/SMX. •Vit A if malnourished •Avoid antidiarrheals	•↑risk seizures, HUS •↑WBC & bandemia
Salmonella	•Poultry & eggs cause ~50% disease. Excreted in stool x 5 weeks	•Incubation 1-3 days, moderate - severe watery diarrhea, fever ~ 38.5-39°C	•Treat infants <3 mos & asplenic patients with ampicillin or TMP/SMX •Avoid antidiarrheals	•Rare: Meningitis osteomyelitis, sepsis •↑ shedding if treated with antibiotic
Yersinia enterocolitica	•Pork, milk, contaminated water	•Acute onset abdominal pain, fever, diarrhea (watery-mucousy)	•↓excretion with antibiotics (Bactrim, tetracycline).	•Mesenteric adenitis mimics appendicitis
C difficile	•Recent antibiotic use	•Mild-severe diarrhea (+/-blood)	•Metronidazole PO	•Vancomycin PO

Abx=antibiotics, HUS=hemolytic uremic syndrome, PO=orally, pt=patient, Rx=treatment, sx=symptoms, TMP/SMX=Trimethoprim-sulfamethoxazole

FAILURE TO THRIVE (FTT)

DEFINITION: No definitive definition exists, consider one of the following:
- Significant weight loss crossing 2 percentile lines on standard growth curves (see section on growth charts & cdc.gov/growthcharts), usually in children < 2 years old.
- Insufficient weight or height gain, especially weight or height <3-5% or weight/height < 85% mean for age
- Differentiate from familial short stature, constitutional growth delay, and small-for-gestational-age infants.

ETIOLOGY

Inadequate Caloric Intake	
Psychosocial problems	*Anatomic/neurologic problems*

• Improperly prepared formula
• Inappropriate diet (juice, rice water)
• Poverty leading to food shortage
• Food phobia following choking
• Inadequate breast milk production
• Neglect/abuse
	• Cleft palate, micrognathia, macroglossia
	• Poor suck/swallow coordination from:
	  Hypotonia, hypothalamic tumor
	  ("diencephalic syndrome"),
	  neuromuscular weakness (botulism,
	  myasthenia gravis, muscular dystrophy)

Improper Calorie Utilization	
Malabsorption	*Metabolism defects*
• Cow's milk protein allergy • Celiac disease • Inflammatory bowel disease • Pancreatic insufficiency • Bacterial overgrowth	• Inborn error of metabolism • Growth hormone deficiency • Glycogen storage disorders

Increased Caloric Needs	

• Hyperthyroidism
• Congestive heart failure
• Prematurity
• Malignancy
• Chronic liver disease
	• Chronic infection: HIV, tuberculosis
	• Renal disease: Renal tubular acidosis,
	  chronic renal failure, Fanconi syndrome
	• Chronic lung disease: Bronchopulmonary
	  dysplasia, asthma, cystic fibrosis

- **Diet history**: Breast fed vs formula, formula preparation & storage, volume consumed (frequency/duration of feeds), maternal diet if child breast fed, solid food, other liquids (juice, rice water, teas). Assess caregiver's understanding of problem.
- *Neurologic exam*: Especially suck/swallow coordination, latch, and tone
- Plot current and previous growth parameters on appropriate growth chart
- 72-hour food diary crucial to assessing sufficiency of diet

TREATMENT

- **Caloric supplementation** based on severity of FTT and underlying diagnosis:
  Infants: "Non-organic" FTT infants need ~150% recommended daily calories for "catch-up" growth. Mix formula >20 kcal/oz or add fortifier to breast milk.
  Toddlers and older children: Dietary log. Consider high calorie foods such as butter, whole milk, cheese, peanut butter, "instant" breakfast drinks, *PediaSure®*
- Follow weight weekly initially, then monthly as weight velocity increases
- Hospitalize severe FTT to initiate feeding and evaluate parent-child interaction

CELIAC DISEASE (Gluten-Sensitive Enteropathy)

Definition: Sensitivity to gluten (after prolonged gluten exposure to wheat, rye, barley containing foods)→ small intestine inflammation→ malabsorptive state. Common: 1:250 in United States, 10-15% 1° relatives affected, all ethnicities, genetic marker is HLA-DQ2, ♀:♂ = 3:2

Clinical Features: Commonly presents between late infancy→2-3 years of age.

Symptoms	Signs	Lab findings
•Failure to thrive	•Irritability	•Anemia (↓iron and/or folate)
•Diarrhea	•Pallor	•Hypoalbuminemia
•Muscle wasting	•Dropping growth	•↑ Alkaline phosphatase &
•Hypoproteinemia	percentiles	↓serum calcium (↓vitamin D)
•Post-prandial emesis	•Pruritic rash on	•Coagulopathy (↓vitamin K)
•Anorexia	elbows/knees/back	•Serologic markers (see below)

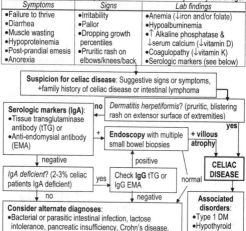

Suspicion for celiac disease: Suggestive signs or symptoms, +family history of celiac disease or intestinal lymphoma

Serologic markers (IgA):
•Tissue transglutaminase antibody (tTG) or
•Anti-endomysial antibody (EMA)

— no → *Dermatitis herpetiformis?* (pruritic, blistering rash on extensor surface of extremities)

— + → **Endoscopy** with multiple small bowel biopsies

yes → **CELIAC DISEASE**

+ villous atrophy →

negative ↓

IgA deficient? (2-3% celiac patients IgA deficient)

yes → Check **IgG** tTG or IgG EMA

positive ↑

normal →

negative ↓

no ↓

Consider alternate diagnoses:
•Bacterial or parasitic intestinal infection, lactose intolerance, pancreatic insufficiency, Crohn's disease, cystic fibrosis, eosinophilic gastroenteritis

Associated disorders:
•Type 1 DM
•Hypothyroid
•IgA deficiency

TREATMENT

Life-long gluten-free diet: Refer to specialist (gastroenterologist and dietician)
•Avoid ALL wheat, rye, barley containing foods. Oats likely safe. Corn, rice ok.
•Expect ↓diarrhea, vomiting & irritability within weeks. Hypocalcemia, rapid weight loss or no response to gluten-free diet may require corticosteroids.
• Lactose intolerance common. Vitamin, mineral, & iron supplements if deficient

Gastroenterology 2001;120:1522-40.

• ↑risk of non-Hodgkin intestinal lymphoma (normalizes after 5 years gluten-free)
• ↑neurologic conditions: Ataxia, peripheral neuropathy, migraines, & depression

Resources: Celiac Sprue Association: www.csaceliacs.org, www.celiac.nih.gov

HLA=human leukocyte antigen, DM=diabetes mellitus, Ig=immunoglobulin

GASTROESOPHAGEAL REFLUX DISEASE (GERD)

INFANTS

Symptoms: Crying with feeds, arching back, Sandifer syndrome, poor weight gain, apparent life-threatening event [(ALTE) up to 95% have GERD by pH probe[3]]; 67% of infants spit up at 5 months, 21% at 7 months, 5% at 1 year.

Differential: (nonbilious emesis): Pyloric stenosis (projectile emesis, 2 wks-4 mo) formula intolerance, gastroenteritis, tracheoesophageal fistula, obstruction

OLDER KIDS / ADOLESCENTS

Signs & Symptoms: Vomiting, abdominal or chest pain, chronic cough, asthma, pneumonia, sinusitis, eroded tooth enamel, hoarseness.

Differential: H. Pylori ± peptic ulcer disease (PUD), infectious esophagitis (herpes, HIV, candida, cytomegalovirus), eosinophilic esophagitis (usually associated with food allergens, especially cow's milk), corrosive ingestions (including lodged tetracycline or other medication), gastritis, Zollinger-Ellison

DIAGNOSIS: Often clinical, and empiric treatment may be considered.
► 24 hour pH probe is the gold standard (larynx + esophagus sensors): reflux index measures cumulative time with pH< 4; + if > 12% (< 1 yr old); > 6% (> 1 yr old)
► Barium swallow/ esophagram [sensitivity (20–60%)/ specificity (64–90%)[3]]; good initial study in kids with dysphagia and for detecting anatomic anomaly.
► Esophageal radio nucleotide reflux scan (scintiscan) can help identify aspiration.
► Endoscopy with biopsy and laryngoscopy (normal does not exclude GERD)
► Bronchoscopy with bronchoalveolar lavage (looking for lipid laden macrophages)

TREATMENT: (medications not needed if only symptom in *infant* is spitting up)

	Lifestyle changes	*H₂ Receptor Antagonists*	*Proton Pump Inhibitors (PPI's)*
Infants	Thicken feeds, "Reflux formulas"	► Ranitidine 4-10 mg/kg/ day divided bid (syrup 15 mg/ mL)	► Lansoprazole*: <10kg: 7.5 mg PO daily 10-20 kg: 15 mg daily >20 kg: 30 mg daily
Older Kids	Avoid caffeine, mint, chocolate, citrus, fatty foods, large meals. Weight loss if indicated.	► Ranitidine 4-10 mg/kg/ day divided bid (max 300mg /day); (capsule 150 mg or 300 mg; granules150 mg) ► Famotidine 1 mg/kg/ day divided bid (Tabs 10, 20, 40 mg; Chewable: 10mg)	► Lansoprazole*: <30 kg: 15mg PO daily >30 kg: 30 mg PO daily (Caps: 15 mg, 30 mg; Granules: 15, 30 mg) ► Omeprazole*: 1.4 mg/kg/day
► Metoclopramide 0.4 mg/kg/ day divided qid may be a treatment option, however efficacy not well documented and possibility of dystonic reactions exists.			

* PPI's not approved for kids < 1 year old. Best before breakfast (bid dosing if nocturnal or extraesophageal symptoms). ↓ symptoms in first 2 weeks. Consider study to confirm GERD if use > 4-6 weeks. Treatment for 3-6 months (possibly longer) likely safe.

Ped Dosage Handbook 9th Ed; J of J Peds 146(3):S3-12; Ped Clinics North America Apr 2003;50(2):487-502

PRE-PARTICIPATION PHYSICAL EXAM

Goal: Identify potentially life-threatening conditions, identify & treat musculoskeletal injuries, plan to prevent new injuries and treat chronic medical conditions (asthma), and suggest appropriate sports for medically-complex children. Can use as opportunity for well-child check (immunizations, social history/counseling).

Sudden death: ~1/200,000 athlete years, ♂>♀, generally no prior symptoms. Generally due to *cardiac condition*: Hypertrophic cardiomyopathy, coronary artery anomalies, arrhythmia, aortic rupture, commotio cordis, myocarditis

HISTORICAL RED FLAGS

Symptoms	Chest pain/tightness, syncope or near-syncope (especially with exertion), dyspnea or wheezing on exertion, palpitations at rest
Medications	Prescribed, performance-enhancing, illicit, over the counter
Past history	Kawasaki disease, rheumatic fever, congenital heart disease, eating disorder, menstrual abnormalities, asthma, hypertension, musculoskeletal injury, loss of function in one of paired organs (eye, testis, kidney), heat-related illness, previous concussion
Family history	Sudden death of relative <50 yrs old (exercise-related, swimming, or driving), Marfan's, long QT syndrome, congenital heart disease

PHYSICAL EXAM RED FLAGS (Focus on cardiac & musculoskeletal exam)

Hypertension	Diastolic murmur	Fixed split S2	≥ Grade III/VI murmur
Organomegaly	Diminished or unequal pulses	Irregular rhythm	Weight <85% ideal for height
Wheezing	Marfan's habitus	Hypermobility	↓ joint range of motion

Condition	Evaluation/treatment options
Cardiac red flag	Limit participation until evaluated by cardiologist with electrocardiogram, Holter monitor, and/or echocardiogram
Exercise-induced asthma	Spirometry, short or long-acting β-agonist 15 min before exercise. Cromolyn or leukotriene modifiers if β-agonist ineffective
Eating disorder	Limit participation at least until menses normalize.
Diabetes mellitus	Pre and mid-exercise snack, or ↓basal insulin (pump). Check glucose q30 min during, and q15 min after exercise.
Stage II hypertension	Limit participation with controlled & cardiology evaluation. Avoid dietary & performance enhancing supplements.
Mitral valve prolapse	OK to participate unless marked regurgitation, history of syncope or arrhythmia, or history of embolic event
Single functioning paired organ	Consider play with restriction (protective gear), or limit sports allowable depending on specific organ involved (testis, eye)
Splenomegaly	Acute: Avoid all sports. Chronic: Limit contact sports.
Fever, diarrhea	Limit play until resolved (↑risk of dehydration & heat illness)
Atlantoaxial instability	Orthopedic evaluation as risk of spinal cord injury

Clinics in Sports Medicine, April 2004; Vol 23(2); Pediatrics 2005; 116: 1558

ANTICIPATORY GUIDANCE FOR PATIENTS WITH SELECT SYNDROMES

Marfan Syndrome: Tall, thin, arachnodactyly, hypermobile joints, ↑arm span-to-height. Autosomal dominant inheritance.

<u>Yearly ophthalmologic examination</u>: Lens dislocation (60%), myopia, strabismus

<u>Aortic root dilation</u>: Yearly echocardiogram; dental prophylaxis if prosthetic valve or residual defect after repair; β blockers slow widening of aorta.

<u>Other complications</u>: Scoliosis, inguinal hernia, spontaneous pneumothorax

Turner Syndrome: Female with short stature, webbed neck, edema of hands/feet, wide-spaced nipples (shield chest), low posterior hairline, cubitus valgus

<u>Genetics</u>: Absence of 2nd X chromosome (45 XO); no association with ↑maternal age or ↑risk of recurrence in future pregnancies; 1 in 2-5000 live births.

<u>Refer</u>: To cardiologist, endocrinologist, geneticist. Renal ultrasound at diagnosis.

<u>Growth failure</u>: Growth hormone therapy when height <5% (usually ~2 years old)

<u>Renal anomalies</u>: Horseshoe kidney, duplicated collecting systems

<u>Delayed puberty</u>: Endocrinologist for estrogen when full height potential reached.

<u>Cardiac problems</u>: Coarctation of aorta, aortic valve/root anomalies, hypertension

<u>Other</u>: Hip dysplasia, hearing loss, hypothyroidism (screen yearly >4 years old)
See: Health Supervision for Children with Turner Syndrome, *Pediatrics* 2003;111:692-702.

Noonan Syndrome: Phenotypically like Turner syndrome. Autosomal dominant, cardiac valve stenosis, equal ♂:♀ prevalence, no chromosomal anomaly.

Williams Syndrome: Supravalvular aortic stenosis, failure to thrive, mental retardation (average IQ = 60), hypercalcemia, characteristic facies, peripheral pulmonic stenosis. Check vision & labs (calcium, electrolytes, thyroid studies)

DiGeorge Syndrome: Deletion of chromosome 22q11 →variable anomalies

<u>Cardiac</u>: Ventricular septal defect, atrial septal defect, Tetralogy of Fallot, transposition of the great vessels. Screening echocardiogram at diagnosis.

<u>Immune</u>: Partial vs. complete thymic hypoplasia leads to variable risk for infection.

<u>Parathyroid</u>: Hypocalcemia in infancy (seizures).

<u>Mid-facial</u>: Cleft lip/palate, typical facies (low set ears, hypertelorism, short philtrum)

Achondroplasia: Autosomal dominant, 75% are new mutations, normal intellect, average adult height = 4 feet. Growth hormone only if proven deficient.

<u>Screen Infants</u>: *Polysomnography*: ↑risk of obstruction and disordered breathing
CT scan craniocervical junction: ↑risk hydrocephalus *(hypotonia, apnea)*
X-rays: Narrow base of skull, large calvaria, lucent proximal femur, trident hands

<u>Children</u>: Yearly hearing screen. Slow motor development due to hypotonia and large head. Plot head circumference at all visits. Otitis media, gastroesophageal reflux, leg bowing, speech & teeth problems common.

<u>Adult</u>: Lumbosacral spinal stenosis with nerve root compression common.
Refer for behavioral health counseling as child/adolescent (↑ risk of depression).
See: Health Supervision for Children with Achondroplasia, *Pediatrics* 2005;116:771-783

DENTAL ISSUES

"TEETHING"	Primary (1°) Teeth Eruption		1° Teeth Exfoliation	Permanent teeth Eruption
	Maxillary	Mandibular		
Central incisor	8-12 mo	6-10 mo	6-7 years	6-7 years
Lateral incisor	9-13 mo	10-16 mo	6-7 years	7-8 years
Canines	16-22 mo	17-23 mo	9-10 years	9-11 years
First molar	13-19 mo	14-18 mo	10-11 years	6 years
Second molar	25-33 mo	23-31 mo	11-12 years	12 years
Third molar				20 years

LATE TEETHING: If no teeth by 18 months, check thyroid, growth hormone, and dental x-rays. Refer to dentist & geneticist (↑risk ectodermal dysplasia)
• Teething rings, frozen wet washcloth, acetaminophen, oral gels for comfort.
• First dental visit at 12-18 months old. Subsequent visits every 6-12 months.

FLUORIDE: Age-based daily fluoride supplementation recommendations

Local water fluoride content	Birth-6mo	6mo-3yr	3yr-6yr	6yr-16yr
<0.3 parts per million (ppm)	0 mg	0.25 mg	0.5 mg	1 mg
0.3-0.6 ppm	0 mg	0 mg	0.25 mg	0.5 mg
>0.6 ppm	0 mg	0 mg	0 mg	0.25 mg

>2 ppm: Consider alternate drinking water to prevent fluorosis in children ≤ 8 yrs
•Fluoride varnish: Replaces oral supplementation. ↓ risk of fluorosis.

FLUOROSIS: *Know local water fluoride content   MMWR Aug 17,2001;50(RR14):1-42
•Opaque white staining, or brittle, pitted enamel from excess fluoride during tooth development (<24 months old for the central incisors, ≤8 years old for all teeth).
•Fluoride toothpaste: Avoid in children <2 yrs. Children <6 years, pea-sized drop

TRAUMA	Complete exam (teeth, gums, lips, jaw, bite) crucial	
pulp necrosis: Toothache, pain with palpation, discoloration, ↑mobility		
Injury Type	Definition	Referral
Avulsion	Tooth out of socket (>1 hr poor prognosis): Leave primary teeth out. Reimplant permanent teeth ASAP. Store in isotonic solution (milk, under parent's tongue). Rinse (not scrub) prior to reimplantation.	Immediate
Concussion	Non-mobile, normal appearing; Support structure injury	Routine
Subluxation	Lateral movement/loose tooth from injury to support structures. May require splinting.	24-48 hrs
Intrusion	"Pushed in". X-rays needed to evaluate socket.	Immediate
Extrusion	Displaced out from socket. Rx: Realign & splint	ASAP
Fracture type	Definition	Referral
No pulp exposed	Only hard tissue (enamel, dentin, cementum) involved. Rx: Cap/dressing applied to protect tooth.	ASAP
Complicated: Pulp exposed	Often bleeding from central core of tooth. May require pulpotomy/pulpectomy.	24 hours
Root fracture	Mobile crown loosely attached to tooth. Intraoral radiographs needed. Rx: Splint and pulp therapy.	immediate

LEAD POISONING

Epidemiology: Most common heavy metal poisoning. Lead is still used in batteries, car radiators, electrical solder, and foreign made toys & candies.

Toxicity: Fetuses and children < 6 years old at greatest risk. Symptoms appear at varying levels, and there probably is no such thing as a "safe" lead level.

System	Acute toxicity	Chronic toxicity
Nervous system	Fatigue, malaise, headache, encephalopathy (delirium, ataxia, stupor, seizures, coma)	Same as acute + tremor, ↓libido, irritability, weakness & neuropsychiatric problems
Renal	Fanconi-like syndrome (glucosuria, aminoaciduria, hyperphosphaturia)	Chronic renal insufficiency, interstitial nephritis, proteinuria
Gastrointestinal	Anorexia, nausea, crampy abdominal pain, elevated transaminases	Same as acute toxicity + constipation & weight loss
Hematologic	Anemia (hemolytic) & basophilic stippling	Anemia (hypochromic; microcytic or normocytic)
Rheumatologic	Myalgias & arthralgias	Myalgias, arthralgias & gout
Neuropsychiatric	Behavioral problems, developmental delay, delinquency	

Screening (check local public health recommendations): Universal screening at 12 and 24 months, or risk-based assessment and screening are both acceptable.

High Risk Situations: Lives in or frequently visits (daycare, grandparents) in a home built before 1950. Lives in a home built before 1978 which has been recently remodeled. Sibling with lead poisoning. Exposed to leaded gasoline.

Timing of repeat venous lead level following abnormal screening lab

Screening lead level	CDC	AAP
10-19 mcg/dl	3 months	1 month
20-44 mcg/dl	1 week – 1 month	1 week
45-59 mcg/dl	48 hours	48 hours
60-69 mcg/dl	24 hours	48 hours
>70 mcg/dl	Immediately	Immediately

mcg/dL	Recommended action based on repeat venous lead level
10-14	Repeat within 3 months, evaluate environment for sources, educate†
15-19	Repeat within 2 months, evaluate environment, educate, public health nurse (PHN) referral
20-44	Repeat within 1 month, evaluate environment, educate, PHN referral
45-69	Single drug chelation therapy, and above interventions
≥70	Immediate hospitalization for 2 drug chelation therapy (see below)

†Education: Diet high in calcium, iron, vitamin C & zinc. Limit hand-mouth contact.

Chelation therapy: CDC recommends chelation for all children with blood lead concentrations ≥45 mcg/dL with oral succimer 350 mg/m^2/dose PO q8 hours x5 days, then q12 hours x 14 days; consider repeat courses as necessary. Children with levels ≥70 mcg/dL should be hospitalized and started on IV chelation therapy with CaNa$_2$ EDTA and dimercaprol.   *MMWR Morbid Mortal Wkly Rep* 2000;49:1133–37.

CHILD ABUSE

Definition: Physical, sexual, emotional abuse; or neglect by primary caregiver

Epidemiology	Child-related risk factors	Parent-related risk factors
•~1 million cases/yr •>1400 deaths/yr •45-50% deaths are children <12 months old	•Chronic medical condition •Prematurity: low birthweight •Malformations •Non-biologic relationship to caregiver	•Single-parent household •Alcohol or substance abuse •History of domestic abuse •Low socioeconomic status •Social/physical isolation •Teen parent

Suspicion of Child Abuse

•Contact local child protective services (CPS) and inform parents of concerns
•Consider contacting police if immediate risk to child, or parents are flight risk
•Consider hospital admission to ensure child safety & allow further evaluation

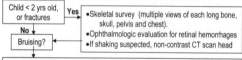

Child < 2 yrs old, or fractures — **Yes** →
•Skeletal survey (multiple views of each long bone, skull, pelvis and chest).
•Ophthalmologic evaluation for retinal hemorrhages
•If shaking suspected, non-contrast CT scan head

No ↓
Bruising? ←

•Consult hematology: CBC, PT, PTT, bleeding time, von Willebrand's studies
•Consult endocrinology or genetics regarding vitamin D and collagen studies

Fractures Suspicious For Child Abuse

•Fracture not consistent with history or developmental skills of child
•Spiral fractures of humerus, femur, or tibia in non-ambulatory child
•Delayed to access care
•Fracture of sternum, scapula
•Posterior rib fracture
•Avulsed clavicle
•Multiple fractures in different healing stages
•Multiple or depressed skull fractures
•Classic metaphyseal lesion (chip fracture)
•Spinal or pelvic fracture without trauma

Brief Differential Diagnosis

Hematologic	Dermatologic	Infectious
•Hemophilia •Idiopathic thrombocytopenia purpura •von Willebrand's disease •Henoch-Schönlein purpura	•Mongolian spots •Vascular malformations •Phytophotodermatitis •Subcutaneous fat necrosis	•Sepsis •Bullous impetigo •Staphylococcal infection

Metabolic	Congenital
•Rickets	•Collagen disorders (osteogenesis imperfecta, Ehlers-Danlos) •Congenital insensitivity to pain

Adapted from Pressel, D, Evaluation of Physical Abuse in Children, *American Family Physician*, May 2000.
CBC: Complete blood count, CT: Computed tomography, PT: Prothrombin time, PTT: Partial thromboplastin time

Links: www.childwelfare.gov, www.preventchildabuse.org, www.pathology.washington.edu/clinical/collagen

CHEST PAIN

EPIDEMIOLOGY: Common complaint, usually benign. ↑risk cardiac disease in pre-adolescents. Majority adolescents have musculoskeletal or psychogenic causes.

DIFFERENTIAL DIAGNOSIS

Idiopathic (35%)	•Generally sharp, brief, intermittent, with or without exercise
Musculoskeletal (30%)	•Costochondritis & chest wall pain (reproducible), slipping rib syndrome (8th, 9th, 10th ribs)
Pulmonary (2-20%)	•Pneumonia, pneumothorax, pleurodynia (coxsackie virus), pulmonary embolus, bronchospasm
Psychological (10-15%)	•Anxiety/panic attack or hyperventilation often associated with dizziness, ↑in adolescent girls, exam normal
Gastrointestinal (5-10%)	•Caustic ingestions, esophageal foreign bodies, esophagitis (tetracycline, "pill" esophagitis, induced vomiting), GERD
Cardiac (2-10%)	•Arrhythmia: Supraventricular tachycardia, PVC •Coronary artery anomalies: Aberrant origin, aneurysms (KD) •Infections: Myocarditis, pericarditis •Structural anomalies: Aortic stenosis, hypertrophic cardiomyopathy, pulmonic stenosis, mitral valve prolapse, coarctation of the aorta, aortic dissection (Marfan's)
Miscellaneous	•Breast mass, acute chest syndrome (sickle cell), zoster

HISTORICAL RED FLAGS

Symptoms	•Exercise induced; radiation to jaw, left arm or back; awakens from sleep; tearing, retrosternal, crushing, recurrent subacute pain, acute onset, hemoptysis, dyspnea, melena, hematemesis
Past history	•Kawasaki disease (KD), congenital heart disease, diabetes
Family history	•Marfan's, Ehlers Danlos, early cardiac death during exercise
Medications	•Oral contraceptives, stimulants, pseudoephedrine, tobacco

DIAGNOSTIC APPROACH

Blood Pressure	Compare to norms for age, gender and height (see pg. 130)
ECG	Obtain for acute onset, pain on exertion, syncope, dizziness, palpitations, cocaine use, associated medical problems Look for ischemia, hypertrophy, strain, arrhythmia
Chest X-ray	Obtain for any red flags or history suggestive of Marfan syndrome, foreign body, tumor or pulmonary pathology
Echocardiogram	Obtain if patient mildly unstable. Consider TEE for rapid diagnosis of aortic dissection and aortic stenosis
Holter monitor	Option in stable patient with history suggestive of arrhythmia
Drug screen	Rule out cocaine, amphetamine use
Cardiac enzymes	If history (♂ ≥ 12, ↑lipids) & ECG suggestive (ST changes)

SUDDEN CARDIAC DEATH: Addition of ECG to pre-participation history and exam may identify ventricular hypertrophy, pre-excitation, or long QT syndrome & ↓relative risk of sudden cardiac death 40-80%. ~2% athletes excluded from play.

ECG: electrocardiogram, GERD: Gastroesophageal reflux disease, KD: Kawasaki disease, PVC: premature ventricular contraction, TEE=trans-esophageal echo   JAMA 2006 Oct 4; 296:1593-601.

DEHYDRATION

ASSESSMENT OF PERCENTAGE DEHYDRATION

Sign/symptom	< 5% (mild)	5-9% (moderate)	>10% (severe)
Fluid deficit	<50 mL/kg	~100 mL/kg	>100 mL/kg
Activity	Normal	Irritable or lethargic	Lethargic or listless
Pulse	Normal	Tachycardic, +/- weak	Thready
Blood pressure	Normal	Normal	Decreased
Capillary refill	Normal	Prolonged	Very prolonged
Mucous membranes	Moist / +tears	Dry / Decreased tears	Dry / No tears
Skin	Normal	Dry, no tenting	Tenting, cold, mottled
Urine	Normal	Decreased UOP, dark	Minimal UOP
Eyes / fontanelle	Normal	Slightly sunken	Markedly sunken

ORAL REHYDRATION SOLUTIONS (ORS)

Solution	CHO (g/dL)	Na (mEq/L)	K (mEq/L)	Base (mEq/L)	Osmolality
WHO/UNICEF	2	90	20	30	310
Pedialyte	3	50	25	30	200
Infalyte	2.5	75	20	30	310
Rehydralyte	2.5	75	20	30	310

INAPPROPRIATE "CLEAR LIQUIDS" FOR REHYDRATION

	CHO (g/dL)	Na (mEq/L)	K (mEq/L)	Base (mEq/L)	Osmolality
Gatorade*	5.8	45.8	12.5		280-340
Apple juice	12	0.4	26	0	700
Chicken broth	0	2	3	3	330
Milk	4.9	22	36	30	260

*Inappropriate CHO:Na ratio impairs water absorption, may ↑osmotic diarrhea

PRINCIPLES OF ORAL REHYDRATION THERAPY

Successful in most children with mild-moderate dehydration

1) Use commercially available ORS, or prepare via instructions @ rehydrate.org
   Rehydration: 50-100 ml/kg PO/NG over 3-4 hours in frequent, small aliquots
   - For each episode emesis or diarrhea, child needs additional fluid as follows:
     - Child <10 kg: 60-120 ml;   - Child >10 kg: 120-240 ml
2) Resume normal diet as soon as possible. Do not restrict diet (avoid BRAT diet)
3) Allow continued breastfeeding. Do not change from, or dilute, standard formula.
4) Avoid unnecessary lab work, antidiarrheal agents, antibiotics & phenothiazines.
5) Consider intravenous 20 ml/kg bolus of normal saline for severe dehydration.
6) IV Ondansetron may ↓emesis. PO zinc may↓diarrhea. Avoid promethazine in
   children < 2 years old and use with extreme caution in older children.

BRAT: bananas, rice, applesauce, toast; CHO: carbohydrate; IV=intravenous; K: potassium; Na: sodium; NG: nasogastric tube; PO: orally; sg: specific gravity; UNICEF: United Nations Children's Fund; UOP: urine output; WHO: World Health Organization

Pediatrics, Mar 1996;97:424–43; *MMWR*, 2003;52(RR-16):1–16; *Pediatrics*, Apr 2002;109:e62

BURNS

Prevention: Smoke detectors; water heater set ≤120° (scald ~85% peds burns)

Depth	Superficial	Partial-thickness	Full-thickness
Color	Pink or red	Superficial=red, deep=yellow	White or brown
Blisters	None	Present	+/- eschar
Pain	Mild – Moderate	Moderate - Severe	Absent
Layers	Epidermis only	Epidermis + dermis	Subdermis
Cause	Sunburn, scald	Flame or scald	Flame, scald
Management	Moisturizers	Debride blisters, see below	Refer

Burns progress over time, have multiple depths of injury within the same wound.

OUTPATIENT MANAGEMENT OF MINOR BURNS

	Bacitracin	Silver sulfadiazine	Mafenide acetate
Indication	Small area; superficial 2nd degree; facial burns	Partial (2nd degree) or full-thickness	Eschar and burns near cartilage
Action	Bacteriostatic	Bactericidal	Anti-pseudomonal
Contra-indication	Allergy to bacitracin	Sulfa allergy; G6PD; infants→kernicterus	Allergy to mafenide acetate
Side effect	Local irritation	Can delay healing & permanently stain	Severe pain; metabolic acidosis

Change gauze bid; change Silver-impregnated absorptive pad q2-3 days

Estimation of body surface area (BSA)	Age (in years)	<1	1	5	10	15
	Head	19%	17	13%	11%	9%
	One thigh	5%	6.5%	8.5%	9%	9.5%
	One leg (below knee)	5%	5%	5.5%	6%	6.5%

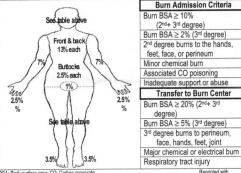

See table above

Front & back 13% each

7%   Buttocks   7%
2.5% each

1%

2.5%   2.5%
%   %

See table above

3.5%   3.5%

Burn Admission Criteria
Burn BSA ≥ 10% (2nd+ 3rd degree)
Burn BSA ≥ 2% (3rd degree)
2nd degree burns to the hands, feet, face, or perineum
Minor chemical burn
Associated CO poisoning
Inadequate support or abuse

Transfer to Burn Center
Burn BSA ≥ 20% (2nd+ 3rd degree)
Burn BSA ≥ 5% (3rd degree)
3rd degree burns to perineum, face, hands, feet, joint
Major chemical or electrical burn
Respiratory tract injury

BSA: Body surface area; CO: Carbon monoxide.

BITES & STINGS

HISTORY & EXAM:
- Break in skin, wound depth, associated symptoms (fever, chills, lymphadenopathy)
- Examine for tendon, joint or bone involvement.

LABORATORY & RADIOLOGY:
- Wound culture if infected, blood culture if febrile or systemically ill.
- Plain radiographs as indicated to look for fractures or joint injury.
- Consider computed tomography (CT) for infants & children with bites to head.

TREATMENT:
- Tetanus prophylaxis for all bite victims
- Copious irrigation for all wounds with normal saline.
- Puncture wounds, minor hand/foot wounds, initial care > 12 hours after bite, cat or human bites, or wounds in immunosuppressed patients should not be sutured. These patients should receive antibiotic prophylaxis as below.

Bite Type	Common organism	Treatment of choice
Human	Viridans strep, S. aureus, Strep. sp, Eikenella corrodens (15% of wounds; very destructive)	AM/CL (erythromycin if penicillin allergic) If signs of infection present: Consider admission for IV AMP/SLB, cefoxitin, or PIP/TAZ
Dog	Pasteurella, Staph, Strep	AM/CL, or clindamycin + TMP/SMX
Cat	Pasteurella multocida	AM/CL or cefuroxime axetil
Bat	S. aureus, strep, rabies	AM/CL, rabies prophylaxis
Rat	Streptobacillus moniliformis	AM/CL

AM/CL: amoxicillin/clavulanate, AMP/SLB: ampicillin/sulbactam, PIP/TAZ: piperacillin/tazobactam, TMP/SMX: trimethoprim/sulfamethoxazole   Ann Emerg Med 1999;33:612-36

RABIES: Saliva of infected mammals→viremia→ fatal encephalomyelitis.
- Thorough cleansing of wound with soap + water, or povidone/iodine solution.
- Quarantine animal for observation. If unable to quarantine, consider prophylaxis for bat, raccoon, fox, skunk & dog bites or contact with bat saliva.
- Rabies immunoglobulin: 20 IU/kg infiltrated around wound, with remainder given IM distant from wound.
- Rabies vaccine: 1 ml IM to deltoid on day 0, 3, 7, 14 & 28.   MMWR 1999;48(RR-1):1-.

SPIDER & INSECT BITES

Black Widow	Toxin	Tetanus prophylaxis, no other treatment
Brown Recluse	Toxin	Tetanus prophylaxis, rarely need systemic treatment (Dapsone) or excision
Fire ant	Mechanical	Ice ↓swelling, cleansing to prevent superinfection

BEE STINGS: Remove stinger immediately (↓venom), treat local swelling with ice.
- Treat pruritus with diphenhydramine (1 mg/kg orally 4-5 doses/day).
- *Systemic symptoms* (wheezing, angioedema): Subcutaneous epinephrine (1:1000 solution), 0.01 ml/kg (max 0.3 ml) + diphenhydramine (see anaphylaxis)
- *Severe local or systemic reactions:* Refer to allergist for possible immunotherapy & prescribe EpiPen (>30 kg) or EpiPen Jr. (<30 kg) for emergent use.

APPARENT LIFE-THREATENING EVENT (ALTE)

Episode that is frightening to the observer, characterized by some combination of:
1) Apnea (central, occasionally obstructive)
2) Color change (usually cyanotic or pallid, but occasionally erythematous or plethoric)
3) Marked change in muscle tone (usually marked limpness)
4) Choking or gagging
- In some cases, the observer fears that the infant has died.
- Occur during sleep, wakefulness or feeding.
- Infants are generally greater than 37 weeks gestational age at time of onset.
- Association with Sudden Infant Death Syndrome (SIDS) not clearly defined.
- Should not use terms "Near-miss SIDS" or "Aborted crib death", as this implies relationship between ALTE and SIDS.

HISTORY

- Timing (awake vs asleep, relation to feeding), location (crib, car seat, etc) and position of infant (prone vs supine) during event are crucial.
- Note presence/absence of choking, coughing, vomitus, respiratory effort, tonic/clonic movements & need for resuscitation.

DIFFERENTIAL DIAGNOSIS (50% cases no etiology discovered)

• Gastroesophageal reflux with glottic spasm • Obstructive apnea • Central apnea • Münchhausen by proxy	• Pertussis • Meningitis • Choking	• Abuse • Sepsis • Seizure	• Cardiac arrhythmia • Hypoglycemia (idiopathic or inborn error of metabolism)

Evaluation: Based on likely etiology from careful history & physical exam.
- Strongly consider admission to hospital for observation.
- Check electrocardiogram, basic blood work (glucose, chemistries, complete blood count, urinalysis).
- Other studies to consider: Electroencephalogram, non-contrast CT scan of the head, gastroesophageal junction pH probe, lumbar puncture, skeletal survey.

Pneumogram: May help distinguish between false and true apnea in patients with frequent home alarm. NOT predictive of which infants will die form ALTE/SIDS.

Home Monitoring: Indicated for infants with:
1) Severe ALTE (requiring vigorous stimulation or mouth-mouth resuscitation)
2) Siblings of 2 or more SIDS victims
3) Central hypoventilation
4) Symptomatic preterm infants
- After 2-3 months of home monitoring, may discontinue monitoring infants who do not require vigorous stimulation or resuscitation. Do NOT need "negative" pneumogram to discontinue monitoring.

1986 National Institutes of Heath Consensus Development Conference on Infantile Apnea and Home Monitoring, Pediatrics, 79: 292-299, 1987

SUDDEN INFANT DEATH SYNDROME (SIDS)

"Sudden death of infant less than 1 year of age, which is unexplained by history and in which a thorough postmortem evaluation fails to demonstrate an adequate cause of death."

▶ *"Thorough postmortem"* includes:
- Autopsy
- Review of clinical history
- Review of death scene

▶ 3rd leading cause of infant mortality (#1 congenital anomalies, #2 prematurity)
▶ 90% occur between 1-6 months of age.

Incidence	Differential Diagnosis	Red flags for abuse
•1 death/1800 births •Rare in first week of life or after 6 months	•Infection: sepsis, meningitis •Arrhythmia: SVT, long QTc •Congenital heart disease •Metabolic disorder •Child abuse	•> 6 months old •Previous familial SIDS •Simultaneous twin SIDS •Blood in nose or mouth •Unclear/changing story

SVT: Supraventricular tachycardia

RISK FACTORS

Maternal	Infant	Environmental	Other
•Age < 20 •Low SES •Tobacco use •Poor/late PNC •Unmarried •Illicit drug use	•Prematurity •SGA •Prone sleeping •♂:♀ = 60:40 •Multiple births •Age 2-5 months	•Winter (65-75%) •Soft bedding •Warm temp •Tobacco smoke	•Previous SIDS in family •Absence of breast feeding

PNC: Prenatal care, SES: Socioeconomic status, SGA: Small for gestational age

PREVENTION

▶ After *"Back To Sleep"* campaign SIDS rates dropped ~ 50%
▶ Avoid *"unsafe"* sleep conditions:
- Soft bedding (sofa, water bed, sheepskin)
- Covered head (no pillows, loose blankets/crib bumpers)
- Side sleeping (infants frequently role prone)
- Shared bed (especially obese & drug/alcohol abusing parents)

▶ **Pacifier**: Offer infant pacifier with naps and nighttime sleep, but do not replace if it falls out. Initiate only after breastfeeding well established.
▶ **Home Monitoring** of patients with apnea & apparent life threatening events **does not** predict or prevent future SIDS. Use may be justified in prolonged apnea of prematurity.

*The *benefit of prone position may outweigh risk of SIDS* in infants with specific conditions such as severe gastroesophageal reflux, upper airway anomalies, and premature infants with respiratory distress.

Pediatrics, 2005;116: 716-723, *Pediatrics* 1992;89:112 –1126, *Pediatrics*, Apr 2003; 111:914-917

FOREIGN BODIES (FB)

INGESTION

Symptoms	•Asymptomatic •Possible symptoms include gagging, choking, vomiting, dysphagia, drooling, tachypnea, ongoing emesis
Evaluation	•Plain radiographs of neck, chest & abdomen as indicated •If symptomatic despite normal X-rays consider computed tomography, barium esophagram & esophagoscopy (EGD)
Common sites of obstruction	•Thoracic inlet •Gastroesophageal junction •Pylorus (if FB >2 cm wide) •Duodenum (if FB >5 cm long) •Ileocecal valve

Object	X-rays	Esophageal management	Beyond esophagus
Coin	AP: disk Lateral: linear	Urgent removal: EGD or bougie dilator via esophagus	Weekly X-rays, average 4-21 days to pass
Battery	AP: 2 densities Lateral: Step-off of cathode	Urgent removal as mucosal burn occurs <4 hours & leads to fistula, perforation, scarring	Watch & wait. If in stomach ≥3 days, consider removal
Sharp object	May be negative	Urgent removal in esophagus	Watch and wait, follow with X-rays

*Instruct patients to return immediately for fever, emesis, pain, or melena.

ASPIRATION

Peak 1-3 years old, >50% unwitnessed, ~50% diagnosed ≥ 24 hrs after event

•The American Academy of Pediatrics recommends **not giving children unchopped round or firm foods** (hot dogs, gummy or hard candy, meat or cheese chunks, grapes, nuts, raisins, raw vegetables) until > 4 years old.

Symptoms	Choking, gagging, wheezing, chronic cough, recurrent pneumonia
Exam	•Most often normal •Can have ↓breath sounds, stridor, drooling, cough
Evaluation	•Obtain AP, lateral and inspiratory/expiratory films •Lateral decubitus films (in lieu of inspiratory/expiratory films) may show air trapping & failure to compress lung on side with FB when dependent. >50% X-rays normal despite presence of FB.
Treatment	•Heimlich maneuver or back blows as appropriate •Rigid bronchoscopy: Consider in symptomatic patients or if high clinical suspicion, even if x-rays negative

EAR: Bead, earring, cotton swab, insect. Attempt irrigation, removal with forceps, or magnet (for metal FB). Bleeding and pain common and make removal difficult.

NOSE: Beads, food, tissue, etc. Removal with forceps, alligator clamps. Can pass Foley catheter beyond FB, inflate balloon, and carefully pull back to remove FB. Some risk of aspiration with attempted removal of FB deep in nose.

OFFICE EMERGENCY PREPAREDNESS

Essential airway equipment

Oxygen	Tank + flow-meter, or in-wall delivery
Bag-valve + reservoir	Child (450 ml) & adult (1000 ml) sizes
Bag-valve mask	Infant, child & adult sizes
Suction equipment	Portable or in-wall system + suction tips
Oral airway	Sizes 00-5

Recommended miscellaneous equipment

Arm board/splint	Butterfly needles (18-25g)	Cervical collar	Nebulizer
Cardiac backboard	Emergency drug sheet	Gauze, tape	Defibrillator

Optional equipment

Nasogastric tube (10 & 16 Fr)	Laryngoscope + blades	Intraosseous needle
Endotracheal tubes (3.0-6.5)	Feeding tube (5 & 8 Fr)	Normal saline (500ml)

Recommended medications

Epinephrine 1:1000 & 1:10,000	Dexamethasone	Antibiotics (ceftriaxone)
Albuterol (0.5% or 0.083%)	Dextrose: 25 or 50%	Diphenhydramine

Optional Medications

Atropine	Naloxone	Sodium bicarbonate	Diazepam or lorazepam
Charcoal	Fosphenytoin	Racemic epinephrine	Phenobarbital

HENOCH-SCHÖNLEIN PURPURA (HSP)

Pathology	•Autoimmune IgA-mediated vasculitis
Epidemiology	•♂:♀ 2:1; ↑incidence in children 6 months-6 years old
Symptoms	•Arthritis/arthralgia: Large joints, lower extremities •Abdominal pain: Colicky, bloody stool, emesis
Signs	•Purpura: Palpable, over buttocks & lower extremities •Edema: Scrotal edema common
Differential	•Meningococcemia, rickettsial infection, septic arthritis
Lab analysis	•CBC (normal or ↑platelets); UA (10-20% may have hematuria and/or proteinuria); baseline creatinine & coag studies
Duration	•Days to weeks; most resolve by 4 weeks
Complications	•Nephritis: <1% kids with HSP go on to end-stage renal disease. Monthly urinalysis for 6 months after diagnosis. Refer to nephrologist for persistent proteinuria/hematuria. •Intussusception: Ileoileal > ileocecal. Ultrasound for diagnosis. Surgical reduction for ileoileal, barium/air enema for ileocecal
Treatment	•Non-steroidal anti-inflammatory drugs (ibuprofen, naproxen) or acetaminophen for joint pain •Corticosteroids: Controversial; may ↓duration of arthritis & abdominal pain. Does not prevent recurrence or nephritis.
Recurrence	•1/3 of patients will have recurrence

UA: urinalysis   *Arch Dis Child 2005;90:916-20, Curr Opin Pediatr 2005;17:695-702*

KAWASAKI DISEASE (KD)

- *Vasculitis* of small→medium sized blood vessels resulting in acute febrile illness
- Associated with coronary artery (CA) aneurysms in 20-25% untreated children
- ↑risk CA aneurysm if ♂, patient <1 yr old, fever ≥14 days, or sodium < 135 mEq/L

ETIOLOGY & EPIDEMIOLOGY:
- Unknown trigger, probably post-viral infection; no known person-person spread
- ↑risk in Asians; ♂:♀=1.5:1; peak age ~24 months; 80% KD patients < 5 years old
- Occurs in "mini-epidemics", 1% patients have family history of KD in sibling.

DIAGNOSIS: Fever ≥5 days plus 4 out of 5 of the following for "classic" KD:
- Cervical lymphadenopathy ≥1.5cm diameter, usually unilateral
- Polymorphic rash: Urticarial, maculopapular, scarlatiniform, but NOT vesicular
- Bilateral non-exudative conjunctival injection, often limbic sparing
- Extremity changes: Erythema, edema, periungual desquamation
- Mucous membrane changes: Strawberry tongue, red & cracked lips
- Incomplete KD: Fever and <4 of above findings. More common in children <12 mo
- Associated symptoms: Irritability, jaundice, itching, abdominal pain, vomiting
- Associated signs: Hepatitis, pancreatitis, gallbladder hydrops, aseptic meningitis, urethritis, perineal rash. Rarely acute interstitial nephritis or acute renal failure.

DIFFERENTIAL DIAGNOSIS: Large differential, most common listed below:
- Adenovirus: Endemic upper respiratory infection; fever, cough, conjunctivitis
- Scarlet fever: Group A strep toxin induced illness with pharyngitis, fever, maculopapular "sandpaper" rash, desquamation on palms (along Pastia's lines)
- Epstein-Barr virus (EBV): "Mononucleosis", fever, pharyngitis, rash (especially if treated with amoxicillin), hepatitis, leukopenia
- Stevens-Johnson syndrome: Fever, rash, mucous membrane involvement
- Juvenile idiopathic arthritis (JIA): Arthritis, fever, uveitis

EVALUATION: Baseline echocardiogram & ECG and referral to peds cardiology.
- Elevated erythrocyte sedimentation rate (>40), C-reactive protein (>3 mg/dl)
- Consider viral testing for adenovirus & throat culture for group A streptococcus
- Complete blood count: Anemia; possible thrombocytosis in 2nd week of illness.

TREATMENT: ↓risk coronary aneurysms if treated within 10 days of illness onset.
- IVIG: 2 gm/kg over 10-12 hrs. If fever persists, consider repeat dose in 24-48 hrs.
- Aspirin (ASA): 80-100 mg/kg/day divided qid for 14 days from onset of symptoms (anti-inflammatory), then 3-5 mg/kg daily until follow-up echocardiogram (6-8 wks later) confirmed as normal. Stop ASA for influenza or varicella-like illnesses.
  - Continue low-dose ASA therapy indefinitely if coronary anomalies present.
- Corticosteroids: Remain controversial, but may be useful for KD refractory to IVIG.
- Dipyridamole: Anti-platelet therapy for patients deemed high-risk for thrombosis.

FOLLOW-UP & PROGNOSIS:
- Treatment (IVIG) before 10 days of illness ↓risk coronary artery aneurysm to <5%.
- Repeat echocardiogram at 6-8 weeks and again at 6-12 months.

Circulation 2004;110; 2747-71. 2006 Red Book: American Academy of Pediatrics, pgs: 412-416.

CAR SAFETY SEATS

Seat type	Age/ weight	Comments
Infant only	Up to 20-30 pounds, depending on type	Rear facing until 1 year old and ≥20 pounds
Convertible	~30 pound rear- facing weight limit and 40-65 pound front- facing limit (varies). Ready for booster when reach weight/ height limit, shoulders above strap slots, ears at top of seat; use as long as possible.	Read manufacturer's instructions. Work well for larger infants.
Booster seat	Use until seatbelt fits correctly without booster (4' 9" & 80 pounds; ~ 8-12 yrs old)	Used with safety belt in vehicle.

*Regulations vary by state; these are general guidelines.

▶ Kids are safest in back middle seat (up to age 13). If child has to sit in the front seat, move seat all the way back *and* turn airbag off.
▶ Safety seat should be discarded after crash unless minor accident (for example, the vehicle was driven away, door by safety seat was undamaged, there were no injuries, airbags did not go off, no visible damage to safety seat).
▶ Seatbelt adjustors are not recommended.
▶ Premature infants: Use seat with 5-point harness, no shield. Car seat test for infants < 37 weeks gestation prior to hospital discharge.

RESOURCES FOR PARENTS

▶ http://www.aap.org/family/carseatguide.htm (car seats, weight limits, contacts)
▶ http://www.seatcheck.org, or 1-866 SEATCHECK
▶ nhtsa.dot.gov/people/injury/childps/contacts/ (find help with seat installation)
▶ Children with special needs: Easter Seals 800/221-6827 or Automotive Safety Program 317/274-2977 www.preventinjury.org.
▶ Consumer product safety commission car seat recall information: www.cpsc.org

LACERATIONS

Location	Suture type	Removal	Dermabond®
Scalp	3-4 nylon or staples	7-12 days	Apply 3 layers for low-tension, dry, well-apposing, wounds.
Face	6 nylon	3-5 days	
Body	4-5 nylon	7-14 days	
Arms, legs	4-5 nylon	7-14 days	Avoid use in punctures, mucosal, contaminated, wet, bite, & jagged wounds
Neck	5 nylon	4-6 days	
Hands, feet	4-5 nylon	7-12 days	

•Lidocaine 1%: Maximum 3-4.5 mg/kg (or 0.3-0.45 ml/kg). Effect lasts 1-2 hours
•Bupivacaine 0.25-0.5%: Maximum 0.5 ml/kg. Lasts several hours.
•Lidocaine, epinephrine, tetracaine (LET): Simple face/ scalp wounds; topical; apply to wound for 10-20 minutes. When edges are blanched, wound is numb.

GROWTH

Height prediction: (can use bone age & current height)
♀: mean parental height (inches) – 2.5
♂: mean parental height (inches) + 2.5

Normal growth rates:

0-2 years: average 14 inches (total) 3 years to puberty: 5 cm (2 inches)/ year Puberty: 8 cm (3.1 inches)/ year

SHORT STATURE:

▶ < 5 % ile for age; most pathologic causes have ↓ growth *velocity* (< 5 cm/ year).

Causes:

Genetic, constitutional delay, idiopathic, malnutrition, chronic illness (renal, cardiac, cystic fibrosis, neoplastic), celiac disease, inflammatory bowel disease, endocrine, syndrome (Turner's, Down, Noonan, Russell-Silver, Prader-Willi), intrauterine growth retardation, achondroplasia

Clues to etiology of short stature:

	Growth velocity	Bone age	Weight
Genetic	normal	appropriate	variable
Constitutional delay	normal	delayed	variable
Idiopathic	normal	appropriate	variable
Cushing's	↓	usually normal	↑ for height
Hypothyroidism	↓	± delay	↑ for height
Growth hormone deficiency	↓	delayed	↑ for height
Malnutrition/ chronic illness	variable	variable	↓ for height

Workup: (based on history, growth pattern and exam findings)

Bone age x-rays; CBC; erythrocyte sedimentation rate (ESR); celiac workup; prealbumin/ transferrin; karyotype; thyroid, renal & hepatic function studies; insulin-like growth factor (IGF-1), insulin-like growth factor binding protein (IGFBP-3); consider MRI (tumor/ pituitary abnormality?); sweat chloride

TALL STATURE: Causes include familial, Marfan's Syndrome, Soto syndrome, growth hormone excess, thyrotoxicosis, Klinefelter syndrome, obesity, precocious puberty, Beckwith-Wiedemann syndrome, homocystinuria.

ANEMIA

Normal RBC indices per age (mean & +/- 2 SD)

Age	Hb (g/dl)	Hct (%)	MCV (fL)
Newborn	16.5 +/- 3	51 +/- 9	108 +/- 10
2 wks	16.5 +/- 4	51 +/- 12	105 +/- 19
2 mos	11.5 +/- 2.5	35 +/- 7	96 +/- 19
3-6 mos	11.5 +/- 2	35 +/- 6	91 +/- 17
0.5-2 yrs	12 +/- 1	36 +/-3	78 +/- 8
2-6 yrs	12.5 +/- 1	37 +/- 3	81 +/- 6
6-12 yrs	13.5 +/- 2	40 +/- 5	86 +/- 9
♀>12 yrs	14 +/- 2	41 +/- 5	90 +/- 12
♂>12 yrs	14.5 +/- 1.5	43 +/- 6	88 +/- 10

Differential diagnosis of neonatal anemia:
- Alloimmune hemolysis (ABO or Rh incompatibility)
- Prematurity
- Blood loss
- G6PD or pyruvate kinase deficiency
- Spherocytosis (HS)
- Elliptocytosis

Microcytic	• Fe deficiency: ↑ RDW,↓retic, Mentzer index commonly > 14 • Thalassemia (thal): ↓RDW,↑retic, Mentzer index commonly < 12 (Mentzer index = Mean corpuscular volume/red blood cell count) • Others: Chronic inflammation, lead intoxication
Normocytic (↓retic)	• Transient erythroblastopenia of childhood, aplastic crisis, chronic renal disease, leukemia, Diamond-Blackfan (isolated RBC aplasia)
Normocytic (↑retic)	• *Intrinsic:* HS (↑MCHC), G6PD, pyruvate kinase deficiency, sickle cell disease, Hemoglobin SC disease, Hemoglobin S-β disease • *Extrinsic:* Immune hemolysis, hemolytic uremic syndrome, disseminated intravascular coagulation
Macrocytic	• Folate/vitamin B12 deficiency, Fanconi's anemia, hepatic disease

Fe: iron, G6PD: glucose-6-phosphate dehydrogenase, Hb: hemoglobin, Hct: hematocrit, MCHC: mean corpuscular hemoglobin concentration, MCV: mean corpuscular volume, retic: reticulocyte count

Iron Studies in Hypochromic Microcytic Anemias*

Iron studies (normals)	Iron deficiency	Chronic disease	Lead toxicity
Serum Fe (22-184 mcg/dl)	Low	Low	Normal – high
TIBC (100-400 mcg/dl)	High	Low-normal	Normal
Ferritin (varies by age)	Low	High	Normal - high

*Best test of iron deficiency is response to iron administration regardless of MCV

Quick Reference for Treatment of Iron Deficiency Anemia

- Elemental Fe 6 mg/kg/day leads to ↑retic count in 3-5 d & ↑Hb within 1 week.

Weight	Volume Fe drops (15 mg elemental Fe/0.6 ml)	Weight	Volume Ferrous sulfate elixir (44 mg elemental Fe/5 ml)
5-7 kg	0.6 ml (1 dropper) daily	11-13 kg	4 ml daily
7-10 kg	0.9 ml (1.5 dropper) daily	13-17 kg	5 ml daily
10-13 kg	1.2 ml (2 droppers) daily	17-24 kg	3 ml BID
		24-31 kg	4 ml BID

- If Hb not ↑ in 1 month, consider other etiologies (thalassemia, blood loss).
- Limit milk to ≤16 ounces/day, as calcium inhibits Fe absorption.
- Give supplemental Fe with Vitamin C, which facilitates absorption.

SICKLE CELL DISEASE

Variations of β hemoglobin (Hb) defect: HbSS (65%), HbSC, HbS-β-thalassemia
At diagnosis: Begin antibiotic prophylaxis & folic acid (tables). Refer to hematology.

Penicillin V* (PCN)	Newborn - 3 years			125 mg PO bid
	3 years to at least 5 years old			250 mg PO bid
	Children >5 yrs old: PCN prophylaxis not effective. However, if febrile ≥39°C, should take 250 mg PCN and seek medical care.			
	*Use erythromycin for penicillin allergic patients			

Folic Acid†	< 6 months	6 months-1 year	1-2 years	>2 years
	0.1 mg/day	0.25 mg/day	0.5 mg/day	1 mg/day
†Some centers use 1 mg/day for all ages, others provide no supplementation.				

•Hydroxyurea: May ↓pain crises & acute chest syndrome. Can suppress bone marrow. Hematologist to manage with frequent complete blood cell counts.

Acute Symptoms: Immediate referral	Chronic Problems: refer/screen each visit
Pain, cough, respiratory distress, fever, pallor, fatigue, priapism, dehydration, neurologic symptoms, enlarged spleen	Hypertension, cholelithiasis, retinopathy, avascular necrosis of hip, renal failure, hematuria, cardiomegaly

•**Vaso-occlusive (pain) crisis**: Hydration is key to prevent ongoing sickling & ischemia. Watch for pulmonary edema, especially if history of acute chest syndrome. Control pain with high doses of non-steroidal anti-inflammatory drugs (naproxen, ibuprofen, ketorolac), or narcotics.

•**Acute chest syndrome**: Intrapulmonary sickling leading to chest pain & visible chest x-ray infiltrate. Often develops 2-3 days into pain crisis. May rapidly progress to respiratory failure. Hospitalize for any signs of pulmonary illness.

Health maintenance	< 1 years old	1-5 years old	5-21 years old
Physical exam	q2-4 mos	q3-12 mos	q6-12 mos
CBC & Retic count	q2-4 mos	q6-12 mos	q6-12 mos
Renal, liver function labs yearly; pulmonary & cardiac function tests as indicated			
Transcranial Doppler ultrasound yearly for children 2-20 years old is predictive of future stroke. High risk patients qualify for chronic transfusion.			
Retinal exam yearly once ≥ 8 years old			
Sports participation: Limit high exertion/contact sports & overheating/dehydration			

Immunizations	2, 4, 6 & 12-15 months	2-10 years‡	≥11 years
	Hib & PCV at each visit	MPSV & PPV	MCV4 once
	Yearly influenza vaccine		

Hib=Haemophilus influenza B vaccine, PCV=Pneumococcal conjugate, MCV4=Meningococcal conjugate
‡MPVS4= Meningococcal polysaccharide x1 between 2-10 years, PPV=Pneumococcal polysaccharide x1 at
≥2 years and again 3 years later, q=every. See CDC.gov & MMWR & discuss with pediatric hematologist.

BLEEDING DIATHESES

Type of bleeding	Commonly associated disorder
Mucosal	Platelet disorder, von Willebrand disease
Intramuscular or intra-articular	Clotting factor disorder
Menorrhagia	30% chance of von Willebrand disease (vWD)

MOST LIKELY CAUSES OF PURPURA BY AGE*

Neonatal	Maternal ITP, SLE, drug use, intrauterine infection, TAR syndrome
1-4 years	Idiopathic thrombocytopenic purpura (ITP)
4-7 years	ITP, Henoch-Schönlein purpura

*Always assess for: Trauma, abuse, liver disease, sepsis, vasculitis, renal failure

SLE=systemic lupus erythematosus, TAR=thrombocytopenia-absent radii, Am Fam Phys 2001;64:419-428

LAB ANALYSIS

Check PT, PTT, fibrinogen, bleeding time, platelets. Consult hematologist. Also consider vWD panel, platelet function analysis-100, mixing studies‡, factor levels.

PT	PTT	Bleeding time	Diagnoses
Nl	↑	Nl	Hemophilia (A or B), lupus anticoagulant†
Nl	Nl or ↑	↑	vWD, uremia, medication effect, platelet defect
↑	Nl	Normal (Nl)	Factor VII or vitamin K deficiency; liver disease
↑	↑	Nl or ↑	Factor II, V, X or vitamin K deficiency; liver disease; disseminated intravascular coagulation

Always consider lab error when evaluating coagulation studies. History of menorrhagia in patient or family member highly suspicious of vWD.

Nl=normal, PT=prothrombin time, PTT=partial thromboplastin time, PFA-100=platelet function analysis.
†Lupus anticoagulant: Circulating antibody that prolongs PTT but patient is actually hypercoagulable.
‡Mixing study: Mix patients blood 1:1 with normal serum. In factor deficiency, PT or PTT will correct to normal. If PT or PTT remains prolonged, patient has circulating antibody.

Adapted from Berman et al, Pediatric Decision Making, Mosby 2003.

HYPERCOAGUABLE STATES (CLOTTING DISORDERS)

Inherited	Acquired	Other
Activated protein C resistance (Factor V Leiden mutation) Protein C or S deficiency Prothrombin gene mutation 20210 Antithrombin III deficiency	Immobilization (post-operative, long travel) Estrogen use (OCP) Pregnancy Obesity Trauma	Hyperhomocysteinemia Systemic lupus erythematosus Indwelling central venous catheter Antiphospholipid syndrome

Labs: Complete blood count, d-dimer, fibrinogen, PT, PTT (prolonged with lupus anticoagulant), Protein C, S antithrombin III & homocysteine assays, Prothrombin 20210 & Factor V Leiden gene mutation analysis, anti-cardiolipin antibodies (IgG & IgM), lupus anticoagulant, anti-nuclear antibody

Treatment options (in consultation with hematologist) include: Heparin, low-molecular weight heparin, warfarin, anti-platelet drugs and/or aspirin.

IDIOPATHIC THROMBOCYTOPENIA PURPURA (ITP)

DEFINITION
- Immune mediated destruction of platelets (usually <100,000/mm³) with petechiae, purpura and occasional mucous membrane bleeding. Severe bleeding is rare.

PRESENTATION
- Abrupt onset, usually post-viral illness (1-4 weeks)
- Petechiae and purpura, gingival bleeding, epistaxis, menorrhagia, rare intracranial hemorrhage (ICH)

DIFFERENTIAL DIAGNOSIS
- Leukemia (ALL): Pancytopenia (often mild anemia & leucopenia), lymphoblasts on peripheral smear, bone pain, fever, splenomegaly, hepatomegaly, lymphadenopathy. Isolated thrombocytopenia with no anemia or leukopenia is rarely leukemia. If more than one cell line is low, consider leukemia.
- Aplastic anemia, thrombocytopenia absent radii (TAR) syndrome, connective tissue diseases

LABORATORY FINDINGS
- Severe thrombocytopenia (often < 20,000/mm³) often with large platelets noted on peripheral smear.
- Normal white blood cells, hemoglobin, hematocrit, coagulation studies
- Consider human immunodeficiency virus (HIV) & anti-nuclear antibody (ANA) testing in teens.

TREATMENT OPTIONS
- Optimal treatment is *controversial*. Many experts will treat for platelet count <10,000/mm³, mucous membrane bleeding, or very young children (< 2-3 years old). Watchful waiting appropriate. Mortality without treatment <0.1%.
- Platelet transfusion *does not work*. May have some effect in stopping life-threatening bleed, but platelet count will not increase.
- Intravenous immunoglobulin: 800-1000 mg/kg IV daily for 1-2 days. 95% patients have ↑platelet in 48 hours. Side effects include: Severe headache, fever, chills, aseptic meningitis, allergic reaction.
- Prednisone: Many different regimens used. Consider 3-4 mg/kg/day X 5-7 days, taper off by 21 days (once documented platelet count increasing). *Be sure patient does not have leukemia prior to initiating corticosteroids.*
- Anti-D Ab (*WinRho®*): 50-75 mcg/kg IV in Rh+ patients. Induces hemolysis. ↑Platelets in 24-48 hours. Side effects: Anemia (rarely severe), renal failure.
- Splenectomy: Rarely necessary. Considered in life-threatening bleeds or chronic ITP not responding to other medications.

PROGNOSIS
- Spontaneous resolution in ~50% of patients by 4-8 weeks, 70-80% by 6 months.
- "Chronic ITP" if >6 months duration (should be seeing pediatric hematologist)
- Intracranial hemorrhage (ICH) occurs in < 1% cases. Risks for ICH include head trauma, chronic ITP, & possibly mucous membrane bleeding.

ITP Practice Guideline, Developed by for The American Society of Hematology. Blood 88:3-40, 1996.

IMMUNIZATION SCHEDULE

2007 RECOMMENDED IMMUNIZATION SCHEDULE AGES 0-6 YEARS

	2 mo	4 mo	6mo	12mo	15mo	18mo	2-3 yr	4-6 yr
Hep B[1]	Hep B			Hep B				
Rotavirus[2]	Rota	Rota	Rota					
DTaP[3]	DTaP	DTaP	DTaP		DTaP			DTaP
Hib[4]	Hib	Hib	Hib	Hib				
PCV[5]	PCV	PCV	PCV	PCV			High risk	
IPV	IPV	IPV		IPV				IPV
MMR[6]				MMR				MMR
Varicella[7]				Varicella				Var
Hep A[8]				Hep A (2 doses)				
Influenza[9]				Yearly influenza				
Men[10]								High risk

DTaP: Diphtheria-tetanus-pertussis vaccine; Hep=hepatitis; Hib; Haemophilus influenza B vaccine; IPV=inactivated polio vaccine; Men= meningococcus; MMR=measles- mumps- rubella; MPSV-4= Meningococcal polysaccharide vaccine; PCV= pneumococcal conjugate vaccine; Var= Varicella;

1. Hepatitis B: First dose at birth; second between 1-2 months and 3rd after 24 weeks of age (and > 16 weeks after 1st). Child born to a hepatitis B surface antigen (HBsAg)-positive mother should receive Hep B vaccine and 0.5 mL hepatitis B immune globulin (HBIG) *within 12 hours of birth*. If HBsAg status is unknown, must determine and give HBIG, if indicated, by 1 week of age.

2. First dose by 6-12 weeks, last dose at < 32 weeks.

3. May give 4th DTaP at 12 months if > 6 months since last dose.

4. If *PedvaxHIB®* or *Comvax®* given at 2 & 4 mo, dose at 6 months NOT NEEDED.

5. Trade name: *Prevnar*. Final dose at > 12 months of age. Certain high-risk groups (cochlear implant, functionally or anatomically asplenic, sickle cell disease, HIV) should get PCV (if 24-59 months old) and/ or pneumococcal polysaccharide vaccine (PPSV; if > 2 years old) separated by at least 2 months.

6. Second dose may be given before age 4 years if > 4 weeks since 1st dose and both doses after age 12 months.

7. May give 2nd dose at <4 years old if >3 months since 1st dose & both doses at > 12 months of age.

8. 2 doses should be 6 months apart.

9. All kids 6-59 months and close contacts of 0-59 month olds. Must be 6 months old for trivalent inactivated vaccine (TIV); 0.25 mL for 6-35 months, 0.5 mL if > 3 years. 2 doses for any child receiving for the first time and < 9 years old [4 weeks apart for TIV and 6 weeks apart for intranasal live, attenuated influenza vaccine (LAIV, *FluMist®*)]; LAIV=0.25 ml to each nostril in patients >5 years old.

10. Kids > 2 years old with terminal complement deficiency, asplenia (anatomic or functional), or other high-risk groups. [meningococcal conjugate vaccine (*Menactra®*) used in children ≥ 11 years old]

* Adapted from CDC.gov: Recommended Immunization Schedule for Person Aged 0-6 years United States 2007; Department of Human Health Services and Centers for Disease Control. www.cdc.gov

IMMUNIZATIONS CONTINUED

RECOMMENDED IMMUNIZATION SCHEDULE: AGES 7-18 YEARS

	7-10 years	11-12 years	13-18 years
Tdap[1]		Tdap	*Tdap catch-up*
HPV[2]		HPV (x 3)	*HPV catch-up*
Meningococcal[3]	MPSV4 (↑risk)	MCV4	*Catch-up*
Pneumococcal	*High risk groups should get pneumococcal polysaccharide*		
Influenza[4]	*↑risk or in contact with ↑groups.*		
Hepatitis A[5]	*Catch-up*		
Hepatitis B[6]	*Catch-up*		
Polio[7]	*Catch-up*		
MMR[8]	*Catch-up*		
Varicella[9]	*Catch-up*		

"Catch-up": implies that vaccine should be administered if child did not receive the immunization at the routinely recommended age. See next page for catch-up immunization schedules.

1. Two available formulations in United States: *BOOSTRIX®* (Minimum age =10 years) & *ADACEL®* (minimum age=11 years); give to kids ≥ 11 years old who have completed primary DTaP series. If received Td booster, preferable to wait 5 years to give Tdap, but may be given at any time if during pertussis outbreak or close contact. Only 1 dose of Tdap needed; subsequent boosters are Td only.
2. Minimum age for HPV=9 years. First dose at 11-12 years old, 2nd dose 2 months later, and 3rd dose 6 months after 1st dose.
3. MPSV4 (meningococcal polysaccharide) minimum age 2 years. MCV4 (meningococcal conjugate) minimum age 11 years; MCV4 (MPSV4 is alternative) routinely recommended at 11-12 years, at high school entry, or entry into college dorm living if not previously vaccinated. Asplenia/ complement deficiency should get MPSV4 if aged 2-10; MCV4 or MPSV4 if ≥ 11 years.
4. May use live, attenuated influenza vaccine (*FluMist®*) if healthy and ≥ 5 years of age; 1 dose if prior vaccination; 2 doses (1 month apart) if first flu vaccination and < 9 years old.
5. 2 doses, 6 months apart if not given previously.
6. *Recombivax®* licensed for use in kids aged 11-15 years old as a 2-dose series. All other Hep B vaccines require a 3-dose series.
7. If combined primary series includes both OPV and IPV, must get 4 total doses. If all IPV or all OPV primary series, then 4th dose not necessary as long as 3rd dose was given when patient was ≥ 4 years old.
8. 2 doses, separated by 4 weeks, to be given at any visit (> 1 year old).
9. < 13 years: 2 doses, 3 months apart; ≥ 13 years: 2 doses, 4 weeks apart.

HPV=human papillomavirus; IPV=inactivated polio vaccine, MMR=measles-mumps-rubella vaccine; OPV=oral polio vaccine; Tdap=combined tetanus-diphtheria-pertussis vaccine

* Adapted from CDC.gov Recommended Immunization Schedule for Person Aged 7-18 years United States 2007; Department of Human Health Services and Centers for Disease Control.

CATCH-UP IMMUNIZATION SCHEDULE

Catch Up Schedule Age 4 months- 6 years

	Min Age	Minimum interval between doses			
		Dose 1→2	Dose 2→3	Dose 3→4	Dose 4→5
Hep B	Birth	4 weeks	8 weeks (16 wks after 1st)		
Rota	6 wk	4 weeks	4 weeks		
DTaP	6 wk	4 weeks	4 weeks	6 months	6 months[8]
Hib	6 wk	4 –8 weeks[1]	4-8 weeks[2]	8 weeks[3]	
PCV	6 wk	4 –8 weeks[4]	4-8 weeks[5]	8 weeks[6]	
IPV	6 wk	4 weeks	4 weeks	4 weeks[7]	
MMR	1 yr	4 weeks			
Varicella	1 yr	3 months			
Hep A	1 yr	6 months			

Catch Up Schedule Ages 7-18 years

Td/ Tdap	7 yr	4 weeks	8 wks-6 mo[9]	6 months[10]	
HPV	9 yr	4 weeks	12 weeks		

For catch-up information about Hepatitis B, Hepatitis A, IPV, MMR, Varicella, Polio, please see footnotes of IMMUNIZATION SCHEDULE AGES 7-18 YEARS

1. Hib: 4 weeks between doses if 1 dose at < 12 months. 8 weeks between doses if 1st dose at 12-14 months (only 2 doses needed); no further doses needed if first dose at $\geq$15 months of age.

2. Hib: Between doses 2-3: 4 wks if current age < 12 months; 8 wks if first dose at $\geq$12 months and 2nd dose given at < 15 months; no further doses if any dose given at $\geq$ 15 months.

3. Hib final dose: only needed for kids 12 mo-5 years who got 3 doses before age 12 months.

4. PCV doses 1-2: 4 weeks between doses if first dose at < 12 months and current age < 24 months; 8 weeks (final dose) if 1st given at $\geq$ 12 months or currently 24-59 months; no further doses needed if healthy and 1st dose given $\geq$ 24 months.

5. PCV doses 2-3: 4 weeks between doses if currently < 12 months; 8 weeks between doses if currently $\geq$ 12 months.

6. PCV final dose: Only needed for kids 12 mos- 5 yrs who got 3 doses before 12 mos of age.

7. Polio: If combined primary series of both OPV and IPV, must get 4 total doses. If all- IPV or all-OPV primary series, then 4th dose not necessary if 3rd dose given $\geq$ 4 years old.

8. DTaP: 5th dose not needed if 4th dose given > 4 years old. DTaP not indicated for kids > 7 years.

9. Td: 8 weeks between dose 1-2 if 1st dose of DTaP at < 12 months, 6 months between dose 1-2 if 1st dose DTaP at $\geq$ 12 months.

10. Td: 6 months between doses 3-4 if first dose DTaP at < 12 months. Tdap should be used for single dose of primary series if age appropriate (*ADACEL*® min age 11 years, *BOOSTRIX*® min age 10 years). Td should be used for all other doses. Do not use DTaP > 7 yrs.

DTaP=diphtheria-tetanus-acellular pertussis; Hib=Haemophilus influenza B; HPV=human papillomavirus vaccine; IPV=inactivated polio vaccine; MMR=measles-mumps-rubella vaccine; OPV=oral polio vaccine; PCV=pneumococcal conjugate vaccine (Prevnar); Rota=rotavirus vaccine (Rotateq); Td=tetanus-diphtheria booster; Tdap=combined tetanus-diphtheria-pertussis booster

Adapted from www.CDC.gov Recommended Immunization Schedule for Person Aged 0-6 years and 7-18 years United States 2007; *MMWR* January 5, 2007 / 55(51);Q1-Q4

IMMUNIZATIONS

IMPORTANT CONTACTS:
▶ CDC-recommended storage and handling procedures: 404-639-8222.
▶ Vaccine Adverse Event Reporting System (VAERS): phone 1-800-822-7967,
(for patients: 800-338-2382); fax 1-877-721-0366; www.vaers.org; info@vaers.org.
Report adverse reactions or failures even if not certain that it is related to a vaccine.
▶ Vaccine Injury Compensation Program (VICP): May compensate individuals if
injury or death is related to a vaccine routinely recommended by the CDC.
Information: www.hrsa.gov/osp/vicp, 800-338-2382; to file claim: 202-219-9657

IMMUNIZATION PEARLS

Minimum age/ interval between doses	Can vaccinate 4 days before minimum age/interval (except rabies; if rabies postexposure prophylaxis indicated must, adhere to strict schedule)
Immuno-deficiency	Avoid live-attenuated vaccines (MMR, VZV, OPV) in pregnancy, known immunodeficiency (cancer, long-term glucocorticoids)
Mild illness	May vaccinate children with mild illness with or without fever
Previous reaction	May give vaccine to those who have had previous mild-moderate local reaction. Avoid DTaP if seizure or inconsolable crying with previous dose.
Outbreak	May give MMR to child < 12 months old during measles outbreak (repeat at 12-15 months)
Use of different brand name vaccines	May use different products for different doses. Try to use same DTaP for 1st three doses. May give only 3 doses of *COMVAX®* if used for all doses and final dose is given between 12-15 months of age.
Simultaneous administration	Can give any routine vaccines at the same time, using different syringes and sites (> 1 inch apart)
Unknown vaccination status	Most vaccines given in other countries are adequate quality. Must have written record (not parent recall). If in doubt, re-immunize or check titers.
Blood products	Wait 3-11 months to give MMR or varicella after intravenous immune globulin (IVIG), varicella zoster immune globulin (VZIG), hepatitis B immune globulin (HBIG), blood transfusion. May administer toxoids & inactivated vaccines after blood products.
Palivizumab (Synagis®)	Does not appear to affect response to routine immunizations.
TST / PPD	Place at same time as MMR, varicella or wait 4-6 weeks after. Do not give MMR to person with +TST until treatment initiated.

DTaP=diphtheria-tetanus-pertussis vaccine, MMR=measles-mumps-rubella vaccine, PPD=purified protein derivative, TST=tuberculin skin test, VZV=varicella-zoster vaccine,   www.cdc.gov

IMMUNIZATIONS

VACCINE REACTIONS & ADVERSE EVENTS

Vaccine	Mild reaction	Moderate- severe reaction
DTaP (diphtheria, tetanus, & acellular pertussis)	Fever (25%), local pain/ erythema (25%), swelling of whole arm/ leg (1 in 30) (most common after dose 4 & 5), fussiness (30%), decreased appetite (10%), vomiting (1 in 50)	Seizure (1 in 14,000), 3 + hours of crying (1 in 1000), fever > 105° F (1 in 16,000), anaphylaxis (<1 in a million), long-term seizures, altered level of consciousness, coma, permanent brain damage (RARE)
Hepatitis A	Local pain (20%), headache (1 in 20), decreased appetite (1 in 12), fatigue (3-5 days after vaccine)	Anaphylaxis (very rare)
Hepatitis B	Local pain (10%), mild – moderate fever (12%)	Anaphylaxis (very rare)
Pneumococcal Conjugate	Local pain/erythema (1/4), fever >100.4° F (33%), fever >102.2° F (1/50)	None known to date, but possibility of anaphylaxis always exists
Influenza	Local erythema/ pain, achiness, fever	Anaphylaxis, possible 1-2/ million chance of Guillain-Barré syndrome
Hib	Local pain/ erythema (25%), fever > 101 (5%)	None known
IPV	Mild soreness at site	None known
Meningococcal	Local pain/redness/ fever	? Guillain-Barré Syndrome
MMR	Fever (1 in 6), rash (1 in 20), cervical adenopathy (rare, onset 7-12 days after shot, more common after 1st dose)	Seizure (1/ 3,000), arthralgias (25%) (↑in teen women), ↓platelets (1 in 30,000), parotiditis (rare), anaphylaxis (<1/ million); deafness, coma, seizures, very rare: not clear if result of vaccine
Varicella	Local pain/ erythema (20%), fever (10%), rash (5%) (<1 mo later)	Febrile seizure (< 1 in 1000), pneumonia
Pneumococcal Polysaccharide	Local pain/ erythema < 1 % fever or myalgias	Anaphylaxis
Td	Local pain/ erythema	Anaphylaxis, pain / atrophy at site

* table adapted from CDC/ National Immunization Program website (www.cdc.gov)

Hib=Haemophilus influenza B; IPV=injectable polio vaccine, MMR=measles-mumps-rubella vaccine; OPV=oral polio vaccine; Rota=rotavirus; Td=tetanus-diphtheria booster

IMMUNIZATIONS

VACCINE BRAND NAMES AND CONTENTS

Vaccine	Brand Names
Diphtheria, Tetanus and acellular Pertussis (DTaP)	Infanrix, DAPTACEL
DTaP-Hepatitis B-inactivated poliovirus vaccine (IPV)	Pediarix
Tetanus reduced diphtheria and pertussis booster (Tdap)	Boostrix, ADACEL
Tetanus reduced diphtheria toxoid booster (Td)	DECAVAC, tetanus and diphtheria toxoids adsorbed
Haemophilus influenza B (Hib)	ActHIB, HibTITER
DTaP-Hib	TriHIBit
Hib/ Hepatitis B	Comvax
Hepatitis A	Havrix, Vaqta
Hepatitis B	Engerix-B, Recombivax HB
Hepatitis A - Hepatitis B	Twinrix
Human papilloma virus vaccine	Gardasil
Pneumococcal	Prevnar, Pneumovax 23 (asplenia)
Rotavirus	Rotateq
Meningococcal	Menactra, Menomune-A/C/Y/W-135 (asplenia)
Varicella Zoster	Varivax, Zostavax
Measles, Mumps, Rubella (MMR)-Varicella	ProQuad

Adapted from www.vaccinesafety.edu/thi-table-Oct1606.pdf

DAYCARE / SCHOOL AND INFECTIOUS DISEASES

Routes of Transmission of Common Infectious Agents

Fecal- Oral	Respiratory Droplets	Person to Person
Salmonella, Shigella, Campylobacter, E. Coli, C. Difficile; astroviruses, enteric adenoviruses, hepatitis A, rotavirus, Giardia, Enterobius vermicularis (pinworms)	Pertussis, mycobacterium tuberculosis, Neisseria meningitidis, Strep pneumoniae, group A strep, adenovirus, influenza, human metapneumovirus, measles, mumps, parainfluenza, RSV, parvovirus B19, varicella	Group A strep, Staph aureus, HSV, tinea varicella zoster, lice, scabies, ringworm

Saliva / urine/ blood: Cytomegalovirus, Herpes simplex virus, Epstein-Barr virus |

RSV=Respiratory Syncytial virus; HSV=Herpes Simplex virus; Adapted from AAP Red Book 27th ed, pp132

Children should be **excluded** from childcare or school as follows:

Until symptoms resolved: Lethargy, irritability, shortness of breath, bloody or mucousy stool, ≥ 2 emesis in 24 hours, if the child feels too ill to go, or if staff cannot care for child
Until MD clears: Stomatitis, rash + fever, behavior change, purulent conjunctivitis*
Until 24 hours of treatment completed: Strep pharyngitis, impetigo
Once treatment initiated: Lice, scabies, tinea

*Child with purulent conjunctivitis treated with antibiotic drops may return to school

Duration of school exclusion for specific illnesses

- •1° HSV infection: Until stomatitis resolved
- •E coli/ shigella: Asymptomatic & 2 negative cultures
- •Salmonella: Asymptomatic & 3 negative cultures
- •Pertussis: Until after 5 days of antibiotics
- •Mumps: 9 days after symptoms resolve

- •Measles: 4 days after rash
- •Hepatitis A: 1 week
- •Varicella: all lesions crusted
- •Giardia: No diarrhea x 2 wk
- •Rubella: 6 days after rash starts

▶ No specific recommendations for RSV, Epstein-Barr virus, coxsackie virus, & other viruses. They may shed for weeks to months; consider on individual basis.
▶ Some states may have laws regarding specific communicable diseases

Children should **NOT** be excluded from school/ daycare routinely for:

Parvovirus B19 (most contagious before rash)	HIV	CMV
Warts, molluscum contagiosum	Hepatitis B	Rash (no fever)
Recurrent herpes (labialis or skin*)	Mild respiratory illness	
Non-purulent conjunctivitis (contagious until resolved but may go to school if able to avoid close contact with others and diligent handwashing)		

*Recurrent lesions on exposed surfaces should be covered with clothes or bandage.
CMV=cytomegalovirus, HIV=human immunodeficiency virus
Red Book 27th edition (2006), American Academy of Pediatrics, Elk Grove, ILL

FEVER

▶ Fever defined as ≥100.4°F or 38°C (rectal temp preferred in young children); may consider 39°C as cutoff in older kids (3-36 months) to initiate workup.
▶ Bundling can cause increase skin temperature, but not ↑ rectal temperature.
▶ Report of rectal temp measured at home should be considered valid.
▶ Most fevers have infectious cause, but consider non-infectious causes.
▶ Immunosuppressed kids should be considered on an individual basis.
▶ Febrile children >1 month old with identifiable viral illness (bronchiolitis, varicella, croup, herpangina, gingivostomatitis) have ↓ risk of bacteremia/ serious bacterial infection. Same risk of bacteremia whether or not acute otitis media is present.
▶ Pneumococcal vaccine: ↓invasive pneumococcal disease (all serotypes), ↓ drug resistant pneumococci; serotypes in vaccine cause 82% of invasive disease
▶ Parental preferences may help to guide workup and disposition in some cases.
▶ Any toxic infant/ child should be aggressively worked up and admitted.

Term, previously healthy infant 28-90 days old, T≥ 100.4°F rectally without source, non-toxic appearing, no evidence of focal bacterial infection (skin, soft tissue, bone, joint infection, pneumonia, meningitis)

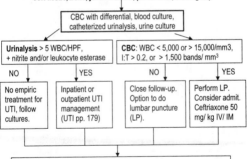

Lumbar Puncture: Should be considered in all patients in this age group. Should be performed if antibiotics will be given. If CSF has > 8 WBC/HPF or positive gram stain, admit for IV antibiotics.

Consider viral swabs for RSV/ influenza if season and clinically indicated. CXR if respiratory symptoms; stool WBC if diarrhea.

CSF: Cerebral spinal fluid, HPF: High-powered field, RSV: Respiratory syncytial virus, UTI: Urinary tract infection, WBC: White blood cell

FEVER CONTINUED

Serious bacterial infections (SBI) in infants and young children

Age	Risk of SBI	Consider workup of:	Other
0-28 days	•12% of febrile neonates have SBI •Respiratory syncytial virus (RSV) positive infants have same risk of SBI	•FOR ALL: CBC, blood culture, catheterized UA and culture, CSF analysis and culture. •Admit for IV antibiotics (ampicillin + either cefotaxime or gentamicin) •CXR, stool WBC if symptomatic	•Consider acyclovir/ HSV studies if: primary maternal infection, prolonged membrane rupture, fetal scalp monitor, vesicles, seizures, CSF pleocytosis, ill.
1-3 months	•Identifiable viral source: 4.2%[1] •No source: 12.3%[1] •Temp >40°C: 38% •RSV positive: 5.5% •RSV negative: 11.7% •Meningitis: 1-4/1000	•CBC, blood culture, •Catheterized UA and culture •Consider lumbar puncture (LP) •CXR / stool WBC if symptoms.	•Serum WBC doesn't reliably predict bacterial meningitis or UTI in this age group. •UTI most common serious bacterial infection.
3-36 months	•"Toxic": 92% •Ill (not well) appearing: 26% •Well-appearing: 3% •0.02% T >39°C and nontoxic have meningococcus •0.1% T >39°C have salmonella	•Consider CBC/ blood culture if high risk.[2] (not routinely indicated if at least 2 doses of PCV-7/ Hib) •Consider catheterized UA→ culture if + LE, nitrites, pyuria, or risk factors[3] •CXR if symptomatic	•Consider bag UA if >1 year old, but catheterize if + •Only catheterized specimens should be cultured. •20% asymptomatic kids with temp >39°C and WBC >20,000 have occult pneumonia

Cath=catheterize, CBC= complete blood count, CSF= cerebrospinal fluid, CXR=chest x-ray,
Hib=Haemophilus influenza vaccine, LE= leukocyte esterase, LP = Lumbar puncture,
PCV=pneumococcal conjugate vaccine, RSV=respiratory syncytial virus, SBI= serious bacterial
infection; T= temperature, UA= urinalysis, WBC= White blood cell

1. Of high-risk infants by lab evaluation (WBC <5000/mm³ or >15,000/mm³, Immature neutrophils: Total neutrophils > 0.2)
2. Unimmunized, meningococcal outbreak, meningococcal contact, fever and petechiae (petechiae more commonly from viral source, especially if well appearing child)
3. Girls with 2 of the following: <12 months old, fever for ≥2 days, temperature ≥39.0°C, Caucasian, no fever source (95% sensitive); all boys < 6 months old & uncircumcised boys < 1 year old.

FEVER CONTINUED

Previously healthy, non-toxic appearing child 3-36 months of age, fever ≥ 39°C without source

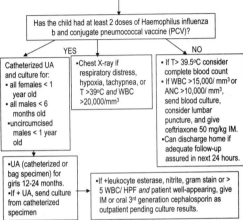

Has the child had at least 2 doses of Haemophilus influenza b and conjugate pneumococcal vaccine (PCV)?

YES

Catheterized UA and culture for:
- all females < 1 year old
- all males < 6 months old
- uncircumcised males < 1 year old

- Chest X-ray if respiratory distress, hypoxia, tachypnea, or T >39°C and WBC >20,000/mm³

NO

- If T> 39.5°C consider complete blood count
- If WBC >15,000/ mm³ or ANC >10,000/ mm³, send blood culture, consider lumbar puncture, and give ceftriaxone 50 mg/kg IM.
- Can discharge home if adequate follow-up assured in next 24 hours.

- UA (catheterized or bag specimen) for girls 12-24 months.
- If + UA, send culture from catheterized specimen

- If +leukocyte esterase, nitrite, gram stain or > 5 WBC/ HPF and patient well-appearing, give IM or oral 3rd generation cephalosporin as outpatient pending culture results.

- Acetaminophen 15 mg/kg/dose every 4-6 hours (do not exceed 5 doses in 24 hours) or ibuprofen 10 mg/kg/dose every 6 hours as needed for fever. Close follow-up warranted. Have patient return if fever persists or condition worsens.

Management of positive blood cultures based on age of patient:
<3 months old: Admit for IV antibiotics
>3 months old: Re-examine. If afebrile and doing well, recheck blood culture and antibiotics as outpatient. If febrile or ill, admit for IV antibiotics.

Baraff LJ, *Ann Emerg Med*, 2000; 36(6):602-14; Ishimine P, *Pediatr Clin North Am*, 2006; 53(2):167-94

TUBERCULOSIS (TB)

▶ 95% of kids <12 years old with TB are acid-fast bacilli (AFB) sputum stain NEGATIVE (secondary to lower AFB burden) and are usually not infectious.

RISK FACTORS FOR TUBERCULOSIS

Urban California, Texas, New York, Illinois, Georgia, Florida, New Jersey, Pennsylvania, minorities, travel to/ born in/ visitor from country with ↑ TB prevalence (country other than US, Canada, Australia, New Zealand, Western Europe); close contact with person with TB or tuberculin skin test (TST) +, contact with adult with HIV/ AIDS, homeless, incarcerated, or substance abuser.

RISK FACTORS FOR PROGRESSION FROM LATENT TO ACTIVE TB

↑ risk if HIV+, malnutrition, diabetes, cancer, chronic renal/ liver disease, immunosuppressive therapy (including steroids), TB infection in past 2 years, < 4 years old, intercurrent viral infections.

DEFINITION OF POSITIVE TUBERCULIN SCREENING TEST
(Based on size of induration and risk factors. Report all + TST to public health.)

> ≥5 mm induration: Close contact with TB, clinical findings suggest TB, immunosuppressed
>
> ≥10 mm induration: Kids < 4 years old, lymphoma, diabetes, chronic renal failure, malnutrition, travel to high risk countries, exposed to ↑ risk adults
>
> ≥15 mm induration: ≥4 years old, no risk factors

▶ All patients with + skin tests should have a chest x-ray (CXR).
▶ Interpret TST in children who received Bacillus Calmette-Guérin (BCG) vaccination the same as non-vaccinated children.

TREATMENT OF LATENT TUBERCULOSIS (TST +, CXR -)

Isoniazid (INH) sensitive	INH 10-15 mg/kg/day MAX 300 mg/ day or 20-30 mg/kg/dose 2x/ week, max 900 mg/ week times 9 months	100 mg, 300 mg tabs; 10 mg/ mL syrup. Monitor liver function.
Isoniazid resistant	Rifampin 10-20 mg/kg/day MAX 600 mg or 10-20 mg/kg/dose 2x/ week x 6 months	150 mg, 300 mg caps Beware: orange urine

▶ Pyridoxine supplementation (1-2 mg/kg/day) is recommended for high-risk patients (HIV, diabetes, renal failure, pregnant, breastfeeding, nutritional deficiency) to reduce the risk of INH-induced peripheral neuropathy.
▶ Active TB (CXR positive or symptomatic) should be treated with a multi-drug regimen, in consultation with TB specialist and public health department.
▶ Newborn should be isolated from mother & evaluated for neonatal TB if mom or other close contact TST+ and symptomatic. If a close contact of the neonate is TST+ but asymptomatic, no special precautions or isolation is necessary.

References: AAP Red Book 2006: Report of the Committee of Infectious Diseases, Tuberculosis pp 678-698; Clin Chest Med 2005; 26(2): 295-312.

MANAGEMENT OF THE TERM NEWBORN

APGAR SCORE (*Performed at 1 & 5 minutes after birth)

	Heart rate	Respiratory effort	Muscle tone	Response to stimuli (catheter in nose)	Color
0	Absent	Absent	Limp	No response	Blue or pale
1	<100	Slow or irregular	Some flexion	Grimace	Body pink, acrocyanosis
2	>100	Crying	Active	Cough/sneeze	Completely pink

Adapted from Apgar, V, *Res Anesth Analg* 1953; 32:260

COMMON NEWBORN INTERVENTIONS (parents can refuse if sign waiver)

Intervention	Medical reasoning
Vitamin K (0.5-1 mg IM) within 1 hour of birth	• Prevents early (birth-2 weeks) and late (2-12 weeks) vitamin K deficiency bleeding (VKDB). • PO vitamin K not recommended: Prevents early, but not late, VKDB (exclusive breastfeeding ↑ risk of vitamin K deficiency) • Very unlikely that IM vitamin K contributes to future leukemia / solid tumors
Gonococcal ophthalmia prophylaxis	• Silver nitrate, tetracycline, or erythromycin acceptable for use in immediate perinatal period. • Occasionally causes chemical conjunctivitis
Hepatitis B immunization	• Decreases vertical transmission of hepatitis B
Newborn screen	• Early discovery of genetic, metabolic, hematologic & endocrine diseases. Provide pamphlet describing tests to new parents.
Hearing screen	• Early diagnosis and intervention with congenital hearing loss has improved outcomes. Refer "failed" tests & infants with ear anomalies for follow-up outpatient audiologic evaluation.

Pediatrics Vol. 112 No. 1 July 2003, pp. 191-192.

CAUSES OF INTRAUTERINE GROWTH RETARDATION (IUGR)

FETAL	PLACENTAL	MATERNAL
• Chromosomal anomalies • TORCH infection • Congenital syndromes • Multiple gestation • Insulin deficiency • Insulin-like growth factor type I deficiency	• ↓Placental weight, surface area or cellularity • Placental infection • Placental infarction • Placental separation • Twin-twin transfusion	• Hypertension • Hypoxemia • Malnutrition • Sickle cell anemia • Drugs (tobacco, alcohol, cocaine, methamphetamine)

• Symmetric IUGR (involves head, length & weight): Often due to early gestational insult/infection (TORCH) or chromosomal anomaly. Generally worse prognosis, with frequent neurologic problems.
• Asymmetric IUGR: More likely late gestational event, such as placental insufficiency. Generally good prognosis.
• IUGR infants may require closer observation as they are at higher risk for hypoglycemia, polycythemia, hyperbilirubinemia, and temperature instability.

TORCH=Toxoplasma, "other" (such as syphilis), rubella, cytomegalovirus, hepatitis, HIV

Modified from Behrman: Nelson's Textbook of Pediatrics, 17th ed, 2004

GENERAL NEWBORN ISSUES CONTINUED

HYPOGLYCEMIA

- Definition: Level at which symptoms become noted, or glucose <40-45 mg/dL in 1st 24hrs of life, glucose <45-50 mg/dL after 24 hrs of life.
- Symptoms: Often asymptomatic. May have jitters, poor feeding, transient cyanosis, apnea, lethargy, convulsions, pallor, high-pitched cry, tachypnea.
- At Risk: Prematurity, maternal diabetes, hypothermia, hypoxia, intrauterine growth retardation, sepsis, small for gestational age (SGA; <2500 g), large for gestational age (LGA; >4000 g) infants.
- Screen: at-risk infants in 1st hour of life. Follow abnormal levels after intervention.
- Treatment: Early bottle or breast feeding. Goal glucose >45 mg/dL. If unable to feed, give 2-3 ml/kg of 10% dextrose in water (D10W) & transfer to intensive care unit for IV glucose infusion 4-8 mg/kg/min.
- Severe or prolonged hypoglycemia may lead to neurodevelopmental problems.
  Pediatrics Vol. 105 No. 5 May 2000, pp. 1141-1145

POLYCYTHEMIA (venous-drawn hematocrit >65%)

- More common at high altitude, in post-term, SGA, LGA, infants of diabetic mothers, delayed cord clamping, hypothyroidism, and numerous syndromes.
- Presents: with plethora (red-purple, ruddy skin color) and signs of hyperviscosity: Feeding problems, lethargy, cyanosis, tachypnea, jitteriness, hyperbilirubinemia, hypoglycemia, thrombocytopenia (if DIC developing)
- Treatment: Partial exchange transfusion (with normal saline) for symptomatic infants. No defined hematocrit criteria for treatment of asymptomatic infants.
  Pediatrics Vol. 78 No. 1 July 1986, pp. 26-30

CLAVICLE & HUMERUS FRACTURES

- Heal remarkably well within 1-4 weeks. Look for brachial plexus injury.
- Immobilization of arm by strapping to chest is generally sufficient.

BRACHIAL PLEXUS INJURY

- Definition: Varying degree of paralysis of arm from lateral traction on head & neck, often seen in macrosomic infants with shoulder dystocia.
- Exam: Arm held adducted, internally rotated, forearm in pronation. Lack of Moro & biceps reflex in affected arm. Severe cases have flaccid paralysis.
- Evaluation: Radiographs to rule out fracture. Consider orthopedic, neurology, and occupational therapy (OT) assessment.
- Treatment: Start range of motion exercises, guided by OT, after ~10 days. Intermittent splinting (arm abducted, externally rotated, supinated, wrist extended) for several hours/day may be indicated as well.
- Natural history: Usually resolves 2-6 mos. 5-15% may require microsurgical repair.
- Bad prognostic indicators for long-term recovery of function include Horner's syndrome (ipsilateral ptosis and miosis), ipsilateral diaphragm paralysis, and complete flaccid paralysis of arm.

GENERAL NEWBORN ISSUES CONTINUED

TRANSIENT TACHYPNEA OF THE NEWBORN

- Signs: Tachypnea, with occasional signs of distress (grunting, retracting) in the first day (or two) of life. Rarely require oxygen. Lungs clear. Thought to be from slow absorption of fetal lung fluid. Possible ↑incidence in planned C-sections.
- Radiographs: Normal, or show hyperinflation with small amount of fluid in fissures.
- Differential diagnosis: Respiratory distress syndrome, meconium aspiration, pneumothorax, persistent pulmonary hypertension of the newborn, choanal atresia

OPHTHALMIA NEONATORUM (acquired during vaginal birth)

Causative agents	Exam Findings	Associated symptoms	Treatment
Chlamydia, N. Gonorrhea*, Staph, strep, Haemophilus influenzae, herpes simplex virus	•Chlamydia: First 10 days of life •Gonorrhea: First 3-5 days; copious purulent discharge; usually bilateral; •Complications: Keratitis, loss of vision, corneal perforation	•Chlamydia: Evaluate for pulmonary involvement. •Gonorrhea can be associated with arthritis, bacteremia, and/or meningitis.	•Chlamydia: Erythromycin 30-50 mg/kg/day PO divided qid •Gonorrhea: •Hospitalize; •Blood, eye, CSF cultures; •Ceftriaxone† 25-50 mg/ kg IM/ IV x 1, •Test for other STI's, treat mom/ partner

STI= Sexually transmitted infections; † Cefotaxime is alternative especially if hyperbilirubinemia.
* Infants born to mothers with known untreated gonorrhea infection should get ceftriaxone 25-50 mg/kg IM x 1 (or cefotaxime). No topical treatment necessary.

DISCHARGE CRITERIA FOR TERM NEWBORNS (38-42 weeks gestation)

- No exam anomalies requiring continued hospitalization
- Open-crib axillary temperature between 36.4-37.5°C
- Social risk factors (drug use, teen mother) have been evaluated
- Parents/caregivers educated in basic newborn care
- If jaundiced, baby has been evaluated and appropriate follow-up scheduled
- If circumcised, minimal bleeding > 2 hours after
- Physician follow-up assured
- Minimum void & stool x 1 each
- Minimum 2 successful feeds
- Maternal hepatitis B and syphilis status known and reviewed
- For infants discharged < 48 hours old, scheduled follow up within 48 hours
- Hearing screen & performed (as mandated by local law)

Adapted from American Academy of Pediatrics, American College of Obstetricians and Gynecologists: Guidelines for Perinatal Care, 5th ed. Elk Grove Village, IL, American Academy of Pediatrics, 2002.

GENERAL NEWBORN ISSUES CONTINUED

NEONATAL VOMITING

- Regurgitation common. Often mucoid or even bloody (blood swallowed at delivery). Consider checking Apt test to differentiate swallowed maternal blood from blood originating from the infant.
- If bilious, consider intestinal obstruction. Make infant NPO (nothing by mouth), obtain urgent upper gastrointestinal series and surgical consultation to evaluate for malrotation, midgut volvulus, sepsis, intestinal atresia, Hirschsprung's disease, or meconium ileus.
- If emesis persists, consider obstruction, sepsis, ↑intracranial pressure, metabolic disorders.

DEVELOPMENTAL DYSPLASIA OF THE HIP

Risk Factors: Family history, female sex, oligohydramnios, breech position, possibly swaddling

Physical Signs

Ortolani	Newborn supine, fingers on greater trochanter and thumb on inner thigh; hip flexed & abducted while lifting anteriorly. "Clunk" is + sign.
Barlow	Newborn supine, legs adducted and posterior pressure placed on knee; clunk or noted movement/ feeling of looseness is + sign.

- *High-pitched clicks are very common and usually inconsequential as long as there are no other red flags (asymmetry of thigh/gluteal folds, leg length or knee height discrepancy, restricted hip abduction), no evidence of looseness, and negative Ortolani & Barlow test.*

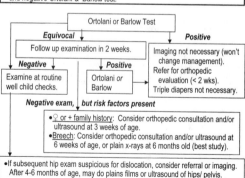

- If subsequent hip exam suspicious for dislocation, consider referral or imaging. After 4-6 months of age, may do plains films or ultrasound of hips/ pelvis.

NEONATAL GROUP B STREPTOCOCCUS (GBS) INFECTION

DEFINITION: ↓incidence with advent of intrapartum antibiotic prophylaxis (IAP).
- Early onset disease (EOD): 80% cases of GBS disease; presents ≤7 days as pneumonia, sepsis, bacteremia or meningitis.
- Late onset disease: 20% of GBS; presents 8 days – 6 weeks, commonly bacteremia & meningitis, occasionally osteomyelitis, septic arthritis, or cellulitis.

DIFFERENTIAL DIAGNOSIS

Pulmonary	Asphyxia, meconium aspiration syndrome, transient tachypnea
Cardiac	Single ventricle physiology, persistent pulmonary hypertension
Metabolic	Hypoglycemia, metabolic disorder, urea cycle disorders
Hematologic	Anemia (blood loss, alloimmune destruction), congenital leukemia
Endocrine	Congenital adrenal hyperplasia, adrenal insufficiency, hypothyroid

RISK FACTORS FOR EOD: Intrapartum antibiotic prophylaxis indicated for vaginal delivery with any of the below criteria.
1. Maternal GBS bacteriuria or urinary tract infection during pregnancy
2. Previous infant with invasive GBS disease
3. Maternal colonization determined by 35-37 week rectovaginal culture
4. Intrapartum fever (temp > 100.4°F) or rupture of membranes > 18 hours
5. Preterm delivery (<37 weeks gestational age)

MMWR. Vol 51 (RR-11) August 16, 2002

Algorithm for management of newborn whose mother received IAP
(adapted from 2006 Red Book: Report of the Committee of Infectious Disease. 27th ed. Elk Grove Village, Ill: American Academy of Pediatrics; 2006)

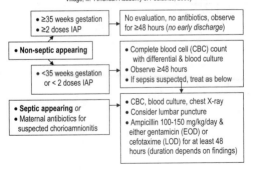

New Ballard Score for Estimating Gestational Age

Score each neuromuscular & physical maturity category, sum the total score and plot on the "maturity rating" table to determine approximate gestational age.

NEUROMUSCULAR MATURITY

NEUROMUSCULAR MATURITY SIGN	SCORE							RECORD SCORE HERE
	-1	0	1	2	3	4	5	
POSTURE								
SQUARE WINDOW (Wrist)	>90°	90°	60°	45°	30°	0°		
ARM RECOIL		180°	140°-180°	110°-140°	90°-110°	<90°		
POPLITEAL ANGLE	180°	160°	140°	120°	100°	90°	<90°	
SCARF SIGN								
HEEL TO EAR								

TOTAL NEUROMUSCULAR MATURITY SCORE

PHYSICAL MATURITY

PHYSICAL MATURITY SIGN	SCORE							RECORD SCORE HERE
	-1	0	1	2	3	4	5	
SKIN	sticky friable transparent	gelatinous red translucent	smooth pink visible veins	superficial peeling &/or rash, few veins	cracking pale areas rare veins	parchment deep cracking no vessels	leathery cracked wrinkled	
LANUGO	none	sparse	abundant	thinning	bald areas	mostly bald		
PLANTAR SURFACE	heel-toe 40-50 mm:-1 <40 mm:-2	>50 mm no crease	faint red marks	anterior transverse crease only	creases ant. 2/3	creases over entire sole		
BREAST	imperceptible	barely perceptible	flat areola no bud	stippled areola 1-2 mm bud	raised areola 3-4 mm bud	full areola 5-10 mm bud		
EYE / EAR	lids fused loosely: -1 tightly: -2	lids open pinna flat stays folded	sl. curved pinna; soft; slow recoil	well-curved pinna; soft but ready recoil	formed & firm instant recoil	thick cartilage ear stiff		
GENITALS (Male)	scrotum flat, smooth	scrotum empty faint rugae	testes in upper canal rare rugae	testes descending few rugae	testes down good rugae	testes pendulous deep rugae		
GENITALS (Female)	clitoris prominent & labia flat	prominent clitoris & small labia minora	prominent clitoris & enlarging minora	majora & minora equally prominent	majora large minora small	majora cover clitoris & minora		

TOTAL PHYSICAL MATURITY SCORE

SCORE

Neuromuscular _____
Physical _____
Total _____

MATURITY RATING

SCORE	WEEKS
-10	20
-5	22
0	24
5	26
10	28
15	30
20	32
25	34
30	36
35	38
40	40
45	42
50	44

GESTATIONAL AGE (weeks)

By dates _____
By ultrasound _____
By exam _____

Reference
Ballard JL, Khoury JC, Wedig K, et al: New Ballard Score, expanded to include extremely premature infants. J Pediatr 1991; 119:417-423. Reprinted by permission of Dr Ballard and Mosby—Year Book, Inc.

Fetal-Infant Growth Chart for Preterm Infants

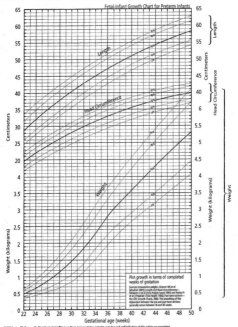

Fetal-Infant Growth Chart for Preterm Infants

Plot growth in terms of completed weeks of gestation

Sources: Intrauterine weight—Kramer MS et al (pediatrics 2001), Length and Head circumference—Niklasson A et al (Acta Pediatr Scand 1991) and Beeby PJ et al (J Paediatr Child Health 1996). Post term portion—the CDC Growth Charts, 2000. The smoothing of the disjunction between the pre and post term sections generally occurs between 36 and 46 weeks.

Gestational age (weeks)

| Name | | | | | | | | Date of Birth | | | | Record # | | | | |

Date							
Age in Weeks							
Length							
Head Circumference							
Weight							

Size for Gestational Age	
SGA	
AGA	
LGA	

NEWBORN SCREEN

▶ Newborn screen is different in every state. Common disorders that are included are:

Disorder	Follow-up to positive screen	Overview of care of child
Congenital hypothyroidism	•Thyroid stimulating hormone (TSH), free thyroxine (FT4) •Consider ultrasound or uptake scan of thyroid •Thyrotropin-binding inhibitor immunoglobulin if evidence of maternal autoimmune thyroid disease •May need to re-screen premature infants at 2-6 weeks	•L-thyroxine 10-15 mcg/kg/day •Goal thyroxine 10-16 mcg/dl & TSH < 6 mU/L •Followup labs (TSH & FT4) 2-4 weeks after start treatment •1st year of life: Check TSH & FT4 every 1-2 months •1-3 years old: Check labs every 3-4 months or 2-4 weeks after dose change.
Galactosemia	•Examine in office for signs of lethargy, hepatic failure •Quantitative galactose 1-phosphate uridyltransferase (GALT), red blood cell galactose-1–phosphate	•Galactose restriction via galactose free formula (soy-based formula)
Cystic fibrosis (CF)	•Immunoreactive trypsinogen, CF mutation analysis •Sweat chloride (>40 mmol/ L is positive; >30 mmol/ L needs to be followed up)	•Nutritional support •May check fecal elastase and consider pancreatic enzyme & fat soluble vitamin (ADEK) supplements •Pulmonary support
Phenylketonuria	•Quantitative phenylalanine and tyrosine	•Phenylalanine restricted diet •Monitor phenylalanine levels
Sickle cell disease	•Confirm results with hemoglobin electrophoresis, isoelectric focusing, or DNA based methods by 2 months of age. •See section on sickle cell disease pg 103	•Penicillin prophylaxis (start by 2 months old) •Timely immunizations: Pneumococcal and meningococcal •Education •Genetic counseling •Monitor for complications

FT4=free thyroxine; TSH=thyroid stimulating hormone

▶ Other disorders that are commonly screened for include biotinidase deficiency, congenital adrenal hyperplasia, homocystinuria, fatty acid oxidation disorders (MCAD deficiency), maple syrup urine disease, and tyrosinemia.

Newborn Screening Fact Sheets; Pediatrics 2006; 118: 934-963

UNCONJUGATED HYPERBILIRUBINEMIA in TERM and NEAR-TERM INFANTS

•Elevated unconjugated bilirubin with conjugated (dbili) <20% of total bilirubin (tbili)

PATHOPHYSIOLOGY

•Heme from red blood cells (RBC) and myoglobin converted to unconjugated bilirubin, travels to liver bound to albumin. Glucuronyl transferase conjugates to dbili, secreted in bile, eliminated via stool. If infant is not stooling well, dbili is hydrolyzed in the colon and reabsorbed back into the circulation.

RISK FACTORS FOR HYPERBILIRUBINEMIA

• Family history of hyperbilirubinemia, polycythemia, cephalohematoma, prematurity, small for gestational age, East Asian or Native American ethnicity, hypothyroidism, sepsis, asphyxia, significant weight loss, exclusive breast feeding, maternal diabetes mellitus.

ETIOLOGY

Decreased Conjugation

•*Physiologic jaundice*: Diagnosis of exclusion for infants 24 hours - 14 days old. Rise < 5 mg/dl/day, peak usually <13 mg/dl. Presumed causes: Immature hepatic enzymes, ↑RBC volume, ↓RBC survival, recirculation from colon.

•*Breast feeding*: Unconjugated, peaks late (1-2 wks), tbili 12-20 mg/dL, possibly from inhibition of liver enzymes. Resolves with switch to formula for 2 days

•*Glucuronyl transferase defect* (Crigler-Najjar I & II): Jaundice < 24 hrs, rapid rise, may require exchange transfusion.

•*Decreased liver function*: Sepsis, hypothyroidism, hepatitis, galactosemia, glycogen storage disease

Overproduction of Heme

•*Antibody mediated hemolysis*: ABO or Rh incompatibility. Coombs +.

•*Red blood cell membrane defects*: Spherocytosis or elliptocytosis

•*RBC enzyme deficiencies*: Glucose-6-Phosphate dehydrogenase (G6PD) deficiency, pyruvate kinase deficiency (PKD)

•*Extravascular blood collection*: Cephalohematoma, intracranial bleed, hematoma at humerus or clavicle fracture.

Abnormal Excretion or Reabsorption of Bilirubin

•*Obstruction*: Biliary atresia, choledochal cyst, cystic fibrosis, Alagille syndrome

•*Abnormal bilirubin transport mechanism*: Dubin-Johnson & Rotor syndrome

EVALUATION: Check tbili in any jaundiced infant < 36 hours old.

•*Ill-appearing*: Consider sepsis, admit to hospital, IV antibiotics. Measure albumin.

•*Well-appearing*: Besides tbili, consider dbili, complete blood count (with differential and pathology review of peripheral smear), reticulocyte count, blood type, direct Coombs test & catheterized urine specimen for culture. G6PD if poor response to phototherapy or ethnicity suggestive (African American, Mediterranean).

• *Transcutaneous bilirubin monitors* need validation; accuracy ↓in dark-skinned and premature infants, and in those previously exposed to sunlight or phototherapy.

UNCONJUGATED HYPERBILIRUBINEMIA in TERM and NEAR-TERM INFANTS

TREATMENT
- Use *hour*-specific graphs to determine need for intensive phototherapy (see following pages)
- ***Ensure hydration***: Continue breast feeding. Supplement with formula or intravenous fluid if significantly dehydrated or limited maternal milk supply. Follow weight closely.
- ***Intensive phototherapy***: Blue-green spectrum (430-490nm), 30 uW/cm^2, maximize skin exposure (diaper & glasses only). If approaching exchange transfusion levels, line incubator with aluminum foil or white material.

MATERNAL-FETAL ABO INCOMPATIBILITY
- Occurs in 20-25% of pregnancies. However, only 10% cases result in hemolysis.
- Hyperbilirubinemia requiring phototherapy occurs in 10-20% of cases.
- Severe anemia requiring transfusion [hemoglobin 6-7 g/dL or symptomatic (poor feeding, tachypnea)] rarely occurs. Once deemed stable for discharge, outpatient follow-up of hemoglobin and reticulocyte count crucial.

KERNICTERUS (ACUTE BILIRUBIN ENCEPHALOPATHY)
- Unconjugated, unbound bilirubin crosses blood-brain barrier and deposits in basal ganglia and brainstem nuclei. Occurs at lower levels in Rh incompatibility & sepsis.
- Early Signs: Hypertonicity, opisthotonus, retrocollis, high-pitched cry, irritability.
- Late Signs: Poor feeding, inconsolable crying, seizures, severe irritability.
- Prevention: Intensive phototherapy or exchange transfusion prior to onset.
- Consider intravenous immunoglobulin for hemolytic disease if tbili approaching exchange transfusion threshold and not responding to intensive phototherapy.

FOLLOW-UP BASED ON RISK ZONE NOMOGRAM (see chart on next page)

Risk Zone	Schedule follow-up within
Low risk	72 hours
Low intermediate	48-72 hours
High intermediate	24-48 hours
High risk	24 hours

Pediatrics 103:6, 1999

- See guidelines for management of hyperbilirubinemia at www.aap.org. Also see www.bilitool.org for downloadable PDA program.

Hour-Specific Nomogram for Determining Future Risk of Needing Intensive Phototherapy in Term and Near-Term Infants

Subcommittee on Hyperbilirubinemia, *Pediatrics* 2004;114:297-316. Reprinted with permission, American Academy of Pediatrics, Elk Grove, Ill

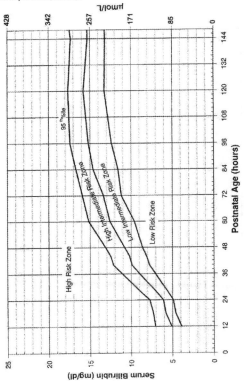

Hour-Specific, Risk-Stratified Guidelines for Intensive Phototherapy in Infants ≥35 wks Gestation

Subcommittee on Hyperbilirubinemia, Pediatrics 2004;114:297-316. Reprinted with permission, American Academy of Pediatrics, Elk Grove, Ill

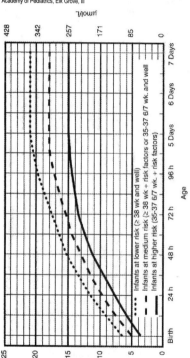

* Use total bilirubin. Do not subtract direct reacting or conjugated bilirubin.
* Risk factors = isoimmune hemolytic disease, G6PD deficiency, asphyxia, significant lethargy, temperature instability, sepsis, acidosis, or albumin < 3.0g/dL (if measured)
* For well infants 35-37 6/7 wk can adjust TSB levels for intervention around the medium risk line. It is an option to intervene at lower TSB levels for infants closer to 35 wks and at higher TSB levels for those closer to 37 6/7 wk.
* It is an option to provide conventional phototherapy in hospital or at home at TSB levels 2-3 mg/dL (35-50mmol/L) below those shown but home phototherapy should not be used in any infant with risk factors.

Hour-Specific, Risk-Stratified Guidelines for Exchange Transfusion in Infants ≥35 Weeks Gestation

Subcommittee on Hyperbilirubinemia, *Pediatrics* 2004;114:297-316. Reprinted with permission, American Academy of Pediatrics, Elk Grove, Ill

▶ Exchange transfusion should be done in a neonatal intensive care unit, and/or in consultation with a neonatologist.

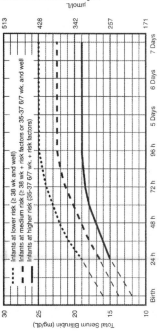

- The dashed lines for the first 24 hours indicate uncertainty due to a wide range of clinical circumstances and a range of responses to phototherapy.
- Immediate exchange transfusion is recommended if infant shows signs of acute bilirubin encephalopathy (hypertonia, arching, retrocollis, opisthotonos, fever, high pitched cry) or if TSB is ≥25 mg/dL (85 μmol/L) above these lines.
- Risk factors - isoimmune hemolytic disease, G6PD deficiency, asphyxia, significant lethargy, temperature instability, sepsis, acidosis.
- Measure serum albumin and calculate B/A ratio (See legend).
- Use total bilirubin. Do not subtract direct reading or conjugated bilirubin.
- If infant is well and 35-37 6/7 wk (median risk) can individualize TSB levels for exchange based on actual gestational age.

HYPERTENSION (HTN)

↑systolic blood pressure (SBP) and/or diastolic blood pressure (DBP) >95% for age, gender & height on ≥3 occasions. Check BP at every visit in children ≥3 years old.

Approximately 1% of children have significant HTN

Pre-hypertension	SBP or DBP 90-95% for age, gender & height, or >120/80
Stage I HTN	SBP or DBP 5 mmHg >95% for age, gender & height
Stage II HTN	SBP or DBP 5 mmHg >99% for age, gender & height
HTN emergency	HTN + acute end-organ dysfunction (severe irritability, seizures, altered mental status, encephalopathy). Immediate referral to intensive care unit.

Technique: Child should be seated & calm for 5 minutes (and off caffeine and other stimulants). Cuff bladder around ≥80% circumference of the extremity.
*Manual BP with auscultation preferred: Stethoscope bell on brachial artery, listen for onset of Korotkoff sounds (SBP) and muffling/disappearance (DBP).
*Too small cuff falsely elevates BP. Too large cuff, minimal effect.

95th Percentile BP Measurements for BOYS by age & height percentile

Age	SBP, mmHg per height percentile			DBP, mmHg per height percentile		
	5th	50th	95th	5th	50th	95th
1	98	103	106	54	56	58
2	101	106	110	59	61	63
3	104	109	113	63	65	67
4	106	111	115	66	69	71
5	108	112	116	69	72	74
6	109	114	117	72	74	76
8	111	116	120	75	78	80
10	115	119	123	78	80	82
12	119	123	127	78	81	83
14	124	128	132	80	82	84
16	129	134	137	82	84	87

95th Percentile BP Measurements for GIRLS by age & height percentile

Age	SBP, mmHg per height percentile			DBP, mmHg per height percentile		
	5th	50th	95th	5th	50th	95th
1	100	104	107	56	58	60
2	102	105	109	61	63	65
3	104	107	110	65	67	69
4	105	108	112	68	70	72
5	107	110	113	70	72	74
6	108	111	115	72	74	76
8	112	115	118	75	76	78
10	116	119	122	77	78	80
12	119	123	126	79	80	82
14	123	126	129	81	82	84
16	125	128	132	82	84	86

Adapted from NHLBI 4th Report on High Blood Pressure in Children, Pediatrics: 114 (2), Aug 2004 Supplement

HYPERTENSION (HTN) CONTINUED

Differential Diagnosis by Age of Patient

<1 yr	Renal artery or vein thrombosis, congenital renal anomalies, coarctation of the aorta, bronchopulmonary dysplasia, central causes (increased intracranial pressure), endocrinopathies [pheochromocytoma, thyroid disease, congenital adrenal hyperplasia (11-hydroxylase deficiency produces aldosterone receptor agonist →hypertension)]
1-6 yrs	Renal parenchymal disease, renal artery stenosis, coarctation of the aorta, Wilms tumor, neuroblastoma, endocrine causes
6-12 yrs	Renal parenchymal disease, renovascular anomalies, endocrine causes (hyperthyroidism)
> 12 yrs	Metabolic syndrome, renal parenchymal disease, endocrine causes

Indications to Check Blood Pressure in a Child < 3 Years Old

Prematurity, neonatal intensive care unit stay, history of umbilical lines, congenital heart disease, urinary tract infection, hematuria, proteinuria, renal disease, urologic malformations, organ transplant, bone marrow transplant, malignancy, illnesses associated with hypertension (neurofibromatosis, tuberous sclerosis), use of drugs known to ↑blood pressure (pseudoephedrine), or family history of congenital renal disease

Symptoms of Hypertension

Patients are often asymptomatic, but may present with irritability, headache, epistaxis, fatigue, shortness of breath, impaired exercise tolerance or impaired academic performance.

3 Phase Approach to the Evaluation of Hypertension

Phase 1	BUN, creatinine, electrolytes, urinalysis, complete blood count, lipid panel, calcium, uric acid, renal ultrasound with Doppler flow, echocardiography, polysomnography, urine toxicology screen
Phase 2	Nuclear medicine renal scan with angiotensin converting enzyme inhibitor, magnetic resonance angiography of the renal vessels, renin profiling, urine catecholamines, plasma and urinary steroids
Phase 3	Renal angiogram/venogram, renal vein renin levels, nuclear med scan of adrenal, caval sampling for catecholamines, aortic angiography

HYPERTENSION (HTN) CONTINUED

TREATMENT OPTIONS

- **Non-pharmacologic:** Useful in all children with pre-hypertension and HTN.
  - Exercise, weight loss, dietary changes: ↓sodium & fats, ↑ fruits & vegetables.
- **Pharmacologic:** Medication class depends on cause of HTN. All drugs ↓BP in short term. Pharmacologic intervention recommended for persistent, symptomatic, or secondary HTN, presence of end-organ damage (left ventricular hypertrophy, renal disease, retinal changes), or comorbid diabetes.
  - Consider baseline echocardiogram and eye exam before initiating therapy.

Common Medications for Hypertension Based on Comorbid Condition

- **Renal parenchymal disease, or any degree of proteinuria:** Angiotensin converting enzyme inhibitor (ACEi)
  Infants: Captopril (0.3-0.5 mg/kg/dose PO tid; max 6 mg/kg/day)
  Children >1 year old: Enalapril (start with 0.08 mg/kg/dose; max 5 mg/day)
  Once ACEi max dose, add angiotensin II receptor blocker.
- **Concomitant migraine:** Beta blocker or calcium channel blocker.
  Metoprolol: 1-2 mg/kg/day PO divided bid, max 4 mg/kg/day (max 640 mg/day)
  Isradipine: 0.05–0.15 mg/kg/day dose given qid (max 0.8 mg/kg/day)
- **Vasculitis/vasoconstriction:** Vasodilators. Consider hydralazine or minoxidil.
- **Sodium retention** (post-infectious acute glomerulonephritis, etc.): Diuretics.
  Hydrochlorothiazide: 1mg/kg/day PO initially, max 3mg/kg/day (max 50 mg/day)
- **Centrally-mediated hypertension:** Clonidine: 5-10 mcg/kg/day PO divided q8-12h. Increase every 5-7 days to 5-25 mcg/kg/day PO div q6h. Max dose 0.9 mg/day.
- Minimal long-term evidence of end-organ protection for any specific class.
- Start single drug therapy at lowest dose, ↑dose until goal BP reached.

Complementary drugs: Once highest recommended dose reached, add 2nd drug from different class
1) Angiotensin converting enzyme inhibitor + diuretic
2) Vasodilator + diuretic or beta-blocker

Ped Clin of North America, 1999(46):2, 235-252

Contraindications to Selected Anti-Hypertensive Medications

- **Angiotensin converting enzyme inhibitor:** Pregnancy, bilateral renal artery stenosis. Watch for increasing serum creatinine and hyperkalemia while on long-term therapy.
- **Beta blockers:** Asthma, diabetes, infants (under age 1)
- **Calcium channel blockers** use is controversial in infants.

Ambulatory Blood Pressure Monitoring (ABPM): Portable outpatient BP device.
- Useful in: "White coat" HTN, severe HTN (with risk of end organ damage), drug resistant HTN, hypotensive symptoms while on therapy.

EVALUATION OF PERSISTENT ATRAUMATIC MICROSCOPIC HEMATURIA

Assuming no vaginal, gastrointestinal, urethral prolapse, hematologic disease or urinary tract infection source

Microscopic hematuria (MH) = >5-10 red blood cells/high powered field

Urine with casts or protein OR UP/Ucr > 0.2 OR family history (FHx) of progressive renal disease

No urine casts or protein, UP/Ucr < 0.2 AND no FHx of progressive renal disease (may have hematuria)

Test: Hearing loss†, creatinine, C3‡, C4, renal ultrasound

Check Urine Ca/Cr (UCa/Cr) ratio and serum creatinine

+ test, deaf or hypertension

Abnormal creatinine

Normal creatinine

Refer to pediatric nephrologist for possible renal biopsy

Ur Ca/Cr >0.2

Ur Ca/Cr <0.2 but FHx of MH

Ur Ca/Cr <0.2, FHx: no MH

24 hour urine for calcium and creatinine, renal ultrasound, consider evaluation for stone

Familial microscopic hematuria

Isolated microscopic hematuria

Possible hypercalciuria

Observe. Recheck urinalysis, creatinine & blood pressure at least yearly. Alport's syndrome may initially present as isolated microscopic hematuria, and only later progress to overt renal disease & deafness.

UP=urine protein, Ucr=urine creatinine, UCa=urine calcium, Ca=calcium, Cr=creatinine
† Alport's syndrome presents with deafness & renal disease
‡ Decreased C3 or C4 associated with postinfectious glomerulonephritis, HIV, systemic lupus erythematosus, hepatitis B, endocarditis, and shunt nephritis

Adapted from Tarascon Pediatric Emergency Pocketbook, 5th edition, Tarascon Publishing, Lompoc, CA   *Pediatrics* 1998; 102:e42

PROTEINURIA

DEFINITION

- Normal protein excretion <100 mg/m^2/day: Limited filtration in glomerulus and reabsorption of filtered low molecular weight proteins (LMWP) by proximal tubule.
- Abnormal protein excretion: >100 mg/m^2/day
- Nephrotic range proteinuria: >1000 mg/m^2/day

EPIDEMIOLOGY

- 5-10% of children have + dipsticks for protein on screening urinalysis (UA); 0.1% have persistent proteinuria.

PATHOPHYSIOLOGY

- <u>Glomerular proteinuria</u>: ↑filtration of large proteins (albumin) due to anatomic changes in glomerulus [minimal change disease (MCD)], and nonpathologic causes: Fever, exercise, orthostatic proteinuria.
- <u>Tubular proteinuria</u>: Failure to resorb normally filtered proteins (β-2 microglobulin, amino acids). Look for associated glucosuria, bicarbonate wasting [proximal renal tubular acidosis (RTA)] & phosphaturia.

LAB IDENTIFICATION OF PROTEINURIA

- <u>Dipstick</u>: Measures albumin, not LMWPs. False +: IV contrast, pH≥8, SG >1.025

Trace	1+	2+	3+	4+
15-30 mg/dL	30-100 mg/dL	100-300 mg/dL	300-1000 mg/dL	>1000 mg/dL

- <u>Sulfosalicylic acid test</u>: Detects all urinary proteins.
- <u>Electrophoresis</u>: Used to detect multiple myeloma.
- <u>Quantitative</u>: 24 hour collection > 100 mg/m^2/day significant, >1000 mg/m^2/day = nephrotic range. Split urine collection to look for orthostatic proteinuria: Negative overnight sample and positive daytime sample diagnostic of orthostatic proteinuria
- <u>Alternative</u>: Spot protein/creatinine (Pr/Cr) ratio (> 0.2 mg/mg = abnormal).

EVALUATION: (see algorithm on next page)

- <u>History</u>: Recent exercise or illness, recent weight gain or edema, change in urine color or frequency, rash, edema, joint pain, family history of renal failure, dialysis, transplantation, or hearing loss.
- <u>Exam</u>: Check blood pressure, weight, edema, heart sounds, arthritis, rash, distal pulses, hearing.

TREATMENT

- <u>Orthostatic & transient proteinuria</u>: Follow-up urine dipstick in 1 year; no treatment recommended.
- Refer persistent proteinuria (Pr/Cr >0.2), or abnormal urinalysis or creatinine to nephrologist, who may consider:
  - <i>Renal biopsy</i>: Pathology may delineate underlying disease.
  - <i>Angiotensin converting enzyme inhibitor</i> may ↓ glomerular protein filtration. Nephrologists ↑dose until blood pressure on low side or side effects noted.
  - <i>Dietary protein restriction</i>: Controversial. Not routinely recommended.

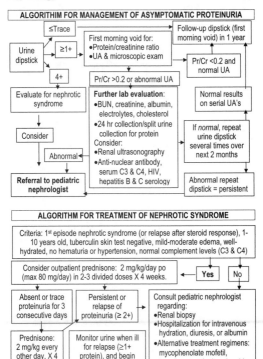

ALGORITHIM FOR MANAGEMENT OF ASYMPTOMATIC PROTEINURIA

Urine dipstick
- ≤Trace → First morning void for:
  - •Protein/creatinine ratio
  - •UA & microscopic exam
- ≥1+
- 4+ → Evaluate for nephrotic syndrome → Consider → Abnormal → **Referral to pediatric nephrologist**

First morning void:
- Pr/Cr <0.2 and normal UA → Follow-up dipstick (first morning void) in 1 year
- Pr/Cr >0.2 or abnormal UA → **Further lab evaluation:**
  - •BUN, creatinine, albumin, electrolytes, cholesterol
  - •24 hr collection/split urine collection for protein
  - Consider:
  - •Renal ultrasonography
  - •Anti-nuclear antibody, serum C3 & C4, HIV, hepatitis B & C serology → **Referral to pediatric nephrologist**

Normal results on serial UA's → If *normal*, repeat urine dipstick several times over next 2 months → Abnormal repeat dipstick = persistent

ALGORITHM FOR TREATMENT OF NEPHROTIC SYNDROME

Criteria: 1st episode nephrotic syndrome (or relapse after steroid response), 1-10 years old, tuberculin skin test negative, mild-moderate edema, well-hydrated, no hematuria or hypertension, normal complement levels (C3 & C4)

Consider outpatient prednisone: 2 mg/kg/day po (max 80 mg/day) in 2-3 divided doses X 4 weeks. → **Yes** | **No**

Yes:
- Absent or trace proteinuria for 3 consecutive days → Prednisone: 2 mg/kg every other day, X 4 weeks. Then off, no taper needed.
- Persistent or relapse of proteinuria (≥ 2+) → Monitor urine when ill for relapse (≥1+ protein), and begin steroids 2 mg/kg/d until urine clear for 3 days, then 2 mg/kg/d every other day with long taper.

No:
Consult pediatric nephrologist regarding:
- •Renal biopsy
- •Hospitalization for intravenous hydration, diuresis, or albumin
- •Alternative treatment regimens: mycophenolate mofetil, tacrolimus, cyclophosphamide, cyclosporine, pulse methylprednisolone

Hogg RJ - *Pediatrics* 2000;105(6):1242-9

- •<u>Diet</u>: Low sodium diet to limit edema. Normalize diet once in remission.

NEPHROTIC SYNDROME (NS) –
see treatment algorithm previous page

- Severe proteinuria resulting in edema, hypoalbuminemia, and hyperlipidemia.
- ↑glomerular permeability → ↑filtration of large proteins (albumin)→ ↑liver synthesis of albumin & lipids

Glomerular Diseases Associated with Nephrotic Syndrome

	Minimal Change Disease	Focal Segmental Glomerulo-sclerosis	Membranous Glomerulo-nephritis	Membrano-proliferative glomerulo-sclerosis (I&II)
Frequency of pediatric NS	75-80%	10-15%	Rare pediatric; ~50% adult NS	~10%
Age of onset	1-10 yrs	2-10 yrs	40-50 yrs	5-15 yrs
♂:♀	2:1	1.3:1	2:1	
Etiology	Idiopathic	Idiopathic, rarely VUR, familial, obesity	Idiopathic, systemic lupus erythematosus, Hepatitis B or C	Systemic lupus erythematosus, Hepatitis C
Hypertension	<10%	>20%	Infrequent	>35%
Hematuria	10-20%	60-80%	60%	80%
Microscopic Pathology	Foot process fusion seen on electron microscopy	Focal sclerosis → global sclerosis	Thickened GBM, subepithelial IgG & C3	Thickened, split GBM. C3 deposits subendothelial.
Steroid response	80-90%	15-20%	Slows progression	Unknown
Prognosis	Very good. Relapse common, ↓ with age	Renal insufficiency: 25% by 5 yrs, 50-80% by 10	Good in children, Adult: 20-30% ESRD	Progressive renal decline, ESRD by 10 yrs common

COMPLICATIONS

- **Infection**: ↑ risk secondary to loss of immunoglobulins, immunosuppressive therapy & ascites. Yearly influenza vaccination important.
  Peritonitis: Streptococcus pneumoniae, gram-negatives (Escherichia coli). Immunize with polyvalent pneumococcal vaccine when in remission & off steroids. **Treat all fevers as potentially life-threatening.**
  Varicella exposure: If non-immune, consider varicella zoster immune globulin (VZIG) within 72 hrs of exposure.
- **Thromboembolism**: (2-5%) ↓protein C & S and ATIII, ↑fibrinogen & platelets.
  Sites: Pulmonary embolus, clot on indwelling catheters, renal vein or sagittal sinus thrombosis
  Prophylactic anti-coagulation: Not recommended, unless previous clotting event. Limit diuresis and avoid furosemide if albumin <2 mg/dl. Use albumin + furosemide if diuresis is critical. Limit use of central indwelling catheters

ATIII=antithrombin III, ESRD=end stage renal disease, GBM=glomerular basement membrane
VUR=vesicoureteral reflux

	HEADACHE (HA)	

Type	Characteristics	Treatment
Migraine without aura (common)	•Frontal/temporal, unilateral or bilateral •Pulsating/throbbing; moderate – severe; ± nausea/ vomiting •Photophobia or phonophobia •≥5 distinct attacks (recurrent) •Lasts 1-72 hours •↑ with activity, light, noise •Peak age: ♂ 7years, ♀ 11 years •↑ risk: Motion sickness, vertigo, sleepwalking or night terrors	Prevention: •Triggers (avoid, if possible): Alcohol, foods*, stress, menses, sleep deprivation, altitude, fasting, medications, exertion • Daily exercise Acute Management: •Rest/ sleep. •Acetaminophen, ibuprofen, or naproxen •Avoid narcotics •Triptans most useful abortive therapy Consider Prophylaxis: •If >4-5 episodes/month
Migraine with Aura (classic)	• Aura in kids may manifest as irritability, malaise, anorexia, pallor • Sensory, motor or visual changes may occur (minutes-hours) • Headache (as above) after aura	
Tension	•Difficult to differentiate from migraine •Usually bitemporal, stabbing •↑ with stress, noise, in afternoon	•↓ Stress •↑ Relaxation •Acetaminophen or ibuprofen as needed.
Exertional	•Occurs with exercise •Migraine variant •Benign	•Daily conditioning may help alleviate HA •Analgesia as needed
Acute Localized	•Sinusitis, myopia, temporomandibular joint problems	•Depends on cause
Acute Generalized	•_Causes_: Systemic infection or disease (lupus), CNS infection, carbon monoxide toxicity, lead poisoning, hypertension, lumbar puncture, hypoglycemia, trauma, cerebrovascular accident. •_Treatment_: Depends on underlying cause	
Chronic, non-progressive headache	•_Causes_: < 6 months post-concussion; stress, psychological issues, chronic daily headache (> 5/week); medication overuse.	•Minimize analgesic use •Biofeedback •Relaxation therapy •Counseling

* Food triggers for migraine: Aged cheeses (tyramine), chicken liver, avocado, nuts, sour cream, yogurt, bananas, monosodium glutamate, ice cream, hot dogs (meats with nitrates), caffeine.

HEADACHE CONTINUED	
Chronic Progressive Headache (↑*frequency* & *severity* with time)	<u>*Causes*</u>: Brain tumor, pseudotumor cerebri, abscess, hydrocephalus, subdural hematoma, arachnoid cysts (large) <u>*Brain tumor headache*</u>: often focal, severe & incapacitating •Persistent vomiting, especially in AM (6-7 am) •Wakes at night/ pain upon awakening; ↑ pain with straining/ Valsalva •Neuro findings# in 85% at 8 weeks after onset of headache <u>*Treatment*</u>: Depends on cause; neuroimage these patients.

papilledema, ataxia, weakness, dysconjugate gaze.

SPECIFIC MIGRAINE SYNDROMES

Hemiplegic	Cannot move one side of body
Ophthalmoplegic	Cannot move eyes
Basilar Type	Dysarthria, tinnitus, ataxia, paresthesias; avoid triptans
Alice in Wonderland	Distortion of body size and proportion
Acute Confused State	Acutely disoriented

MIGRAINE EQUIVALENTS/ RELATED DISORDERS

Cyclic vomiting/abdominal migraine: Recurrent vomiting; unknown cause
Paroxysmal torticollis: Recurrent episodes of dystonic head tilt in kids <1 year old
Paroxysmal vertigo: Recurrent episodes of vertigo

WORKUP:

▶ Headache journal to assess frequency and severity of symptoms.
▶ Consider non-contrast CT if abnormal neuro exam/ focal findings, chronic progressive headache or suggestions of increased intracranial pressure. If questionable CT result, consider MRI.
▶ Consider lumbar puncture if suspect infection or pseudotumor cerebri.

MEDICATIONS USED IN THE TREATMENT OF PEDIATRIC MIGRAINE

DRUG	DOSE	SIDE EFFECTS
Acetaminophen	15 mg/kg/dose; max 4 g/day	Hepatic dysfunction
Ibuprofen	10 mg/kg/dose; max 1.2 g/day	Renal dysfunction
Naproxen	5-7 mg/kg/dose q 8-12 hours	Renal dysfunction
Sumatriptan (Imitrex) •Approved for kids >12 yrs old •Effective in kids ≥ 8 years old •70% effective	• **Nasal:** 5 mg or 20 mg doses; May start with 5mg but most kids > 8 will have more relief from 20 mg. •**SQ:** 6 mg (0.5mL) (dosing not well established; consider 3 mg if < 30 kg; 6 mg if > 30 kg); •**PO:** Not reliable; may re-dose 1 hour later, if needed.	•Dizziness, drowsiness, nausea, tingling, flushing, chest tightness, arrhythmias, diaphoresis. •Avoid in basilar type migraines.
•*Prophylactic options*: Cyproheptadine (2 mg/5 mL; 2-4 mg PO bid), tricyclics antidepressants, valproic acid, gabapentin, topiramate, riboflavin (consult neurologist)		

SEIZURES

CLASSIFICATION:

> _Partial_: One cerebral hemisphere; _Generalized_: Both hemispheres involved;
> _Simple_: Consciousness unaffected; _Complex_: Consciousness impaired;
> _Motor_: Tonic, clonic or tonic-clonic; _Absence_: Blinking/ staring;
> _Status Epilepticus_: Prolonged (> 20-30 minutes) or multiple seizures without
> recovery between episodes.

DIFFERENTIAL DIAGNOSIS: Syncope (+/- convulsive movements), breath-holding spells, atypical migraine, benign myoclonus, tic disorders, reflux/Sandifer syndrome, pseudoseizures, acute dystonic reaction (medication side effect), night terrors

CAUSES OF SEIZURES IN CHILDREN/ ADOLESCENTS

Infectious	Febrile, meningitis, encephalitis, abscess, neurocysticercosis
Toxic	Cocaine/ other street drugs, lead, isoniazid, lithium, tricyclic antidepressants, hypoglycemic agents
Withdrawal	Alcohol, anticonvulsants
Electrolytes	Hypocalcemia, ↓sodium, ↓glucose, ↓magnesium, hyperosmolality
Vascular	Stroke, arteriovenous malformation, hypertensive encephalopathy, traumatic hemorrhage
Structural	Primary brain tumor or metastases, congenital anomalies
Endocrine	Adrenal insufficiency, hypo or hyperthyroidism
Metabolic	Inborn errors of metabolism
Idiopathic	Other causes have been ruled out

WORKUP

<u>Labs</u>: CBC, metabolic panel, and consider toxicology screen. Others based on history/ physical exam.

<u>EEG</u>: For all with afebrile seizure; helps to determine type and recurrence risk.

<u>Lumbar Puncture (LP)</u>: Consider in kids < 6 months old, altered (or not at baseline) mental status, or meningeal signs.
•CT of the head prior to LP if ↑intracranial pressure suspected.

•<u>Imaging</u>: 1/3 of patients will have abnormality on CT or MRI, but only 2% affect further management (usually in patients with focal seizure or other clinical findings).
•_Emergent imaging_ if suspect trauma, ↑intracranial pressure, or if there is a delay in return to baseline, or residual focal deficits.
•_Non-emergent imaging_: Significant cognitive or motor impairment, abnormal neurologic examination, focal seizure (+/ - generalization), child < 1 year old, or abnormal EEG

SEIZURES CONTINUED

TREATMENT (second line or adjunctive treatment in parenthesis)

Partial Seizures	Carbamazepine, valproic acid, oxcarbazepine, lamotrigine, topiramate
Generalized Tonic Clonic	Topiramate, oxcarbazepine, phenytoin, valproic acid, carbamazepine
Juvenile Myoclonic Epilepsy	Valproic acid, (lamotrigine, topiramate, levetiracetam)
Absence	Ethosuximide, valproic acid, and lamotrigine
Rolandic Epilepsy	Gabapentin, carbamazepine, or observation without meds
Lennox-Gastaut syndrome	Topiramate, (lamotrigine: May ↑myoclonic seizures in some patients)
Infantile Spasms	Corticotropin= ACTH, *Acthargel*; (vigabatrin, valproic acid)
Neonatal Seizures	Phenobarbital, phenytoin, (pyridoxine as adjunct)
Febrile Seizures	Rectal diazepam for prolonged seizure

Adapted from: Initial treatment of epilepsy with antiepileptic drugs, *Neurology* 2004(63), Number 4

POSSIBLE SIDE EFFECTS OF ANTIEPILEPTIC DRUGS

Carbamazepine	Weight gain, sedation, neutropenia/agranulocytosis, ↑ liver enzymes, ↑cholesterol
Oxcarbazepine	Headache, hyponatremia, nausea
Lamotrigine	Rash, dizziness, sedation, Stevens-Johnson syndrome
Topiramate	Somnolence, weight loss, nephrolithiasis
Phenytoin	Hirsutism, gingival hyperplasia, drowsiness, cardiac
Valproic acid	Weight gain, thrombocytopenia, ↑liver function tests
Ethosuximide	Aplastic anemia, hiccups, sedation, rash
Phenobarbital	↓Cognitive performance, ↓attention, ↑cholesterol, sedation
Gabapentin	Weight gain, emotional lability, leukopenia

Adapted from *Neurology*, 2004(63), Number 4

NEONATAL SEIZURES

Presentation	May be tonic (sustained posturing), clonic (rhythmic jerking), myoclonic (isolated jerks) or subtle (tongue/ mouth movements, pedaling, swimming, eye movements/ sustained eye deviation)
Differential diagnosis	Sandifer syndrome (arching with gastroesophageal reflux), jittery (flexion and extension duration are the same; in seizure one is longer than the other), benign neonatal sleep myoclonus (sleep only), apnea, startle response
Causes	Hypoxic-ischemic encephalopathy, infection, bleed, electrolyte anomaly, hypoglycemia, anatomic problem, metabolic, genetic

Zupanc ML, *Pediatric Clinics North Am*, 2004; 51(4): 961-78

FEBRILE SEIZURES

(applies to neurologically normal children 6 months- 5 years old)

Incidence: 4% of children 6 months- 5 years old have febrile seizures.
Definition: Seizure associated with fever, but not associated with intracranial infection or other identifiable cause. Usually occurs within the first 24 hours of a fever.

TYPES OF FEBRILE SEIZURES

	Age	Duration	Seizure Type	Episodes
Simple (75%)	6mo-5yr	< 15 min	Generalized tonic-clonic	1 in 24 hours
Complex (20%)	Any	> 15 min	Focal	> 1 in 24 hours

All criteria under "simple" category must be present for seizure to be classified as a "simple febrile seizure". If any characteristic listed under "complex" category is present, then seizure should be classified as "complex febrile seizure".

	Workup	Treatment
Simple	•Identify source of fever. •If mental status returns to baseline, normal neuro exam, and no signs intracranial infection, no specific workup needed. •Consider lumbar puncture in kids < 18 months old, as meningeal signs less reliable in younger patients.	•Reassurance •Antipyretics do not ↓ risk of febrile seizure •Rectal diazepam if prolonged seizure •Oral or rectal diazepam at fever onset may↓ recurrence (if frequent).
Complex	•More in depth workup warranted. •Identify source of fever •Consider lumbar puncture (especially in kids < 18 months old) •Consider electroencephalogram and neuroimaging studies.	•Other medications may be indicated for complex seizures, depending on results of workup.

PROGNOSIS

	Age at first seizure	Recurrence risk	Epilepsy risk
Simple	< 12 months	50%	1-2.4% (↑ with more seizures)
	> 12 months	30%	1% (slightly > general population)
Complex	Higher risk of underlying pathology and developing epilepsy (2-4%)		

AAP Clinical Practice Guidelines Practice Parameter: Long Term Treatment of the Child with Simple Febrile Seizures; Pediatrics 1999 (103)6, pp 1307-1309; Rosman, NP, Colton T, Labazzo J, A controlled trial of diazepam administered during febrile illness to prevent recurrence of febrile seizures. *N Eng J Medicine* 1993; 329: 79-84; Kutscher M, "Febrile Seizures" from www. pediatricneurology.com

MINOR CLOSED HEAD INJURY (CHI)

EPIDEMIOLOGY: >100,000 minor closed head injuries per year in United States.

EVALUATION OF INFANTS < 2 YEARS OLD

High risk: *Imaging* recommended*	Altered mental status, focal neurologic findings, skull fracture (depressed or basilar), seizure, emesis ≥ 5 times, bulging fontanel, loss of consciousness (LOC) ≥1 minute
Intermediate risk: *Consider imaging or observation*	Transient loss of consciousness, scalp hematoma, resolved lethargy/irritability, resolved emesis (3-4 episodes), subacute (>24 hrs) skull fracture, high force mechanism, unwitnessed fall, fall onto hard surface, vague/changing history, child <12 months old
Low risk: *Observation*	Low force mechanism (fall < 3 feet), normal neurologic exam > 2 hours post injury, and child >12 months old

AAP Guidelines, The Management of Minor Closed Head Injury in Children, *Pediatrics*, 1999;104:1407-1415
*Imaging: Non-contrast computed tomography of the head

COMA SCORES

	Points	GCS	Modified Infant Coma Score
Eye Opening	4	Spontaneous	Spontaneous
	3	To voice	To voice
	2	To pain	To pain
	1	None	None
Verbal Response	5	Oriented	Coos, babbles
	4	Confused	Irritable cry, consolable
	3	Inappropriate	Cries to pain
	2	Garbled	Moans to pain
	1	None	None
Motor Response	6	Obeys commands	Normal movements
	5	Localizes pain	Withdraws from touch
	4	Withdraws from pain	Withdraws from pain
	3	Flexion posturing	Flexion posturing
	2	Extension posturing	Extension posturing
	1	No movement	No movement

SPORTS RELATED CONCUSSION

Trauma induced brain injury, which may or may not involve loss of consciousness (LOC). Mimics include dehydration, hypoglycemia, migraine, heat-related illness.

Acute Symptoms	Late Symptoms
LOC, headache, dizziness, emesis, incoordination, impaired physical skills, amnesia, slurred speech, seizures, confusion, unsteady gait	Headache (persistent), depression, disorganization, poor concentration, frustration, emotionality, personality & behavior changes, memory problems

MANAGEMENT: "ABC's" and C-spine precautions for severe injuries

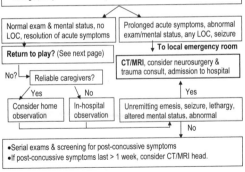

On-site physical & neurologic exam, including field tests of mental status.
- *Orientation*: Person, time & place (current score, opponent, location of game)
- *Attention*: serial 7's or 3's (count backwards from 100), spell word backwards
- *Memory*: Recall 5 words immediately & in 5 min, teacher/coach's name, birthday
- Test speech, visual acuity and fields, extraocular movements, fundus, pupillary reaction, Romberg, finger-nose, heel-toe walk, pronator drift, strength, deep tendon reflexes (DTR's)

Normal exam & mental status, no LOC, resolution of acute symptoms	Prolonged acute symptoms, abnormal exam/mental status, any LOC, seizure

Return to play? (See next page)

To local emergency room

No? — Reliable caregivers?

CT/MRI, consider neurosurgery & trauma consult, admission to hospital

Yes / No

Consider home observation / In-hospital observation

Yes

Unremitting emesis, seizure, lethargy, altered mental status, abnormal

No

- Serial exams & screening for post-concussive symptoms
- If post-concussive symptoms last > 1 week, consider CT/MRI head.

For more information, see: www.cdc.gov/ncipc/tbi/physicians_tool_kit.htm

---
RETURN TO PLAY GUIDELINES for SPORTS-RELATED CONCUSSION

▶ Any abnormality on computed tomography (CT) or magnetic resonance imaging (MRI) terminates season.

▶ Consider imaging for post-concussive symptoms that last >1 week.

Severity	Management (adapted from Cantu & Colorado guidelines)
Grade I •No LOC •Symptoms <15 min	•Examine on sideline every 5 minutes for symptom resolution. •If no symptoms >15 minutes, consider same game return to play. •If symptoms >15 minutes or 2nd closed head injury in same game, no return to play until asymptomatic for 1 week each with rest and with exercise.
Grade II •No LOC •Symptoms >15 min	•Remove from play with frequent on-site examination. •Consider transport to medical facility for imaging. •No play until symptom free for 1 week with both rest and with exercise. •If 2nd grade II concussion, return when symptom-free for 2 weeks with both rest and with exercise.
Grade III •Any LOC	•Remove from play, thorough neurologic evaluation, consider immediate transfer to medical facility for CT or MRI of the head. •Brief LOC (< 1 minute), return to play when symptom free for 1 week each with rest and with exercise. •LOC (> 1 minute), return to play when symptom-free for 2 weeks each with rest and with exercise. •If 2nd Grade III concussion, return when symptom-free for 1 month with both rest and with exercise.

LOC=loss of consciousness   *Clin Sports Med.* 1998 Jan;17(1):45-60, *Colo Med* 1990;87:4

MOVEMENT & BALANCE DISORDERS

- History and exam crucial to diagnosis. Toxicology screen for all with acute onset.
- Consider imaging (MRI, CT head) & neurology consult for all.

Ataxia: Uncoordinated voluntary movement, despite normal strength.
- Disorder of cerebellum. Assess duration. Consider MRI, CT head, EMG, EEG.
- Exam: Abnormal finger-nose, thumb-digit opposition, wide based gait

Acute	• Ingestion • Hydrocephalus • Encephalitis	• Acute post-infectious (particularly varicella) • Guillain-Barré (Miller-Fisher variant) • Stroke • Brain tumor
Chronic	• Friedreich ataxia	• Ataxia telangiectasia • Cerebellar dysgenesis

Vertigo: Sensation of movement (spinning) in relation to surrounding
- Disorder of inner ear (labyrinths, hair cells) or brain stem
- Nystagmus should be present; identify otitis media, neurocutaneous signs
- Consider otolaryngology consult & MRI/CT head for recurrent/chronic symptoms

Acute vertigo	History	Duration	Hearing	Treatment
Benign paroxysmal	Occurs with rapid head movement	10-20 seconds	Normal	Head/neck positioning
Labyrinthitis	No trauma or HA	Days	Often impaired	Meclizine
Perilymphatic fistulae	Due to ↑pressure "pop" at onset	Variable	Fluctuating	Surgical
Labyrinth concussion	Recent trauma	Days	Often impaired	Watch vs surgical
Recurrent vertigo				
Migraine	Headache (HA)	Variable	Normal	See pp. 138
Ménière's disease	Relapsing	Mins/hrs	↓Low-frequency	

Neurologic Clinics 23(3), August 2005

Chorea: Involuntary muscle contractions →twitching & writhing which often "flow" down extremities, causing flinging "ballistic" movement. Suppressed in sleep.

Sydenham's chorea (facial grimacing)	• Associated carditis, arthritis & ↑ASO titer (rheumatic fever) • May respond to valproic acid, haloperidol, prednisone • Lasts weeks to months; 20% recurrence within 2 years
Other causes	• Wilson's disease, Huntington disease, systemic lupus erythematosus • Drugs: metoclopramide, phenothiazines, haloperidol

Dystonia: Involuntary, sustained contraction = slow, twisting of trunk, extremities. Occasionally involves eyelid (blepharospasm) or speech muscles (dysphonia).
- Phenothiazines: May respond to diphenhydramine. Remove inciting medication
- Cerebral palsy: Baclofen, benzodiazepines, botulinum injection
- Familial dystonia: Onset 6-12 years, may be levodopa-responsive

ASO=anti-streptolysin O antibody, CT=computed tomography, EEG=electroencephalogram, EMG=electromyogram, HA=headache, MRI=magnetic resonance imaging

NEUROCUTANEOUS DISORDERS	

NEUROFIBROMATOSIS TYPE 1 (NF1 = von Recklinghausen's disease)

Epidemiology	•Autosomal dominant, 1/4000, though > 50% new mutations
Diagnosis (Need 2 or more)	•≥ 6 café-au-lait spots: Tan-light brown, uniform, sharp-bordered macules (prepubertal >5 mm, postpubertal >15 mm) almost always present by 1 year of life. •≥ 2 neurofibromas •≥ 2 iris hamartomas (seen in only ¼ patients < 6 years old) •1 plexiform neurofibroma •Axillary freckling •Inguinal freckling •1st degree relative with NF-1 •Bony anomaly: Sphenoid dysplasia or thinning of long bones •Optic glioma (15% patients)
Evaluation	•Ophthalmology consult: 20% of gliomas cause vision problems. •Neuroimaging for patients with seizures, precocious puberty, or signs of hydrocephalus. •Blood pressure: Renal vascular stenosis common
Treatment	•Genetic counseling. No other specific treatment.
Differential diagnosis	•McCune-Albright syndrome: Fibrous dysplasia (fractures) & precocious puberty, café-au-lait spots
Resources	http://www.understandingnf1.org/

TUBEROUS SCLEROSIS (TS)

Epidemiology	•Autosomal dominant, ~1/6000-30,000, variable clinical severity
Clinical findings	•Mental retardation (60+%), epilepsy (80+%), begins in infancy, generally severe, may have infantile spasms, cardiac rhabdomyoma ~50% infants, renal angiomyofibroma, autism
Skin findings	•Ash-leaf macule: White, sharp borders, leaf-shaped noted at birth or shortly after, on trunk or extremities. Use Wood's lamp. Solitary hypopigmented patch not uncommon in normal kids. •Adenoma sebaceum: Yellow-red or flesh-colored papules 1-5 mm on face (cheeks & chin) in late childhood. Found in 80-90% TS patients > 4 years old. •Shagreen patch: 1-8 cm, thick, skin-colored lumbosacral plaque •Periungual & gingival fibromas in ~50% patients, pubertal onset
Evaluation	•CT or MRI brain (repeat MRI annually or biannually) •EEG if seizing or tubers present •Renal ultrasound, urinalysis, blood pressure, BUN, creatinine •Echocardiogram in infants (and children with cardiac symptoms) •Neurodevelopmental & psychiatric screening at 2 & 5 years old •Ophthalmology consult
Treatment	•Lamotrigine, carbamazepine, valproate for epilepsy •Sirolimus may cause regression of some hamartomas.
Resources	http://www.tuberous-sclerosis.org/

INFANT NUTRITION

INFANT FORMULAS

Formula Name	Distinguishing factors	Indications
Cow's Milk Based		
With iron Enfamil®, Similac®	•20 calories/ ounce •Protein: whey •Carbohydrate: lactose •Fat: safflower, soy, coconut, palm, sunflower oils. 300 mOsm/ kg	•Standard formula •Normal term infants or infants with no specific nutritional needs
Hypercaloric Enfamil 24® or Similac 24®	•24 calories/ ounce •Other components the same as above except ↑ osmolality (360-380 mOsm/ kg) & ↑ K, Ca, Phos, Cl concentration	•Used for infants with fluid restrictions and/or ↑ calorie requirements
Preterm	•Protein: milk/ whey concentrate •Fat: MCT, soy, coconut oil	•↑ protein concentration and calories for preemies
NeoSure®	•22 calories/ ounce •Carbohydrate: lactose, maltodextrin	
Enfamil Premature®	•24 calories/ ounce •Carbohydrate: corn syrup/ lactose	
Lactose Free	•*Enfamil LactoFree LIPIL, Isomil DF and Similac Lactose Free Advance*	•Lactose intolerance
Reflux Enfamil AR LIPIL®	•20 calories/oz •Protein: nonfat milk •Carbohydrate: lactose/ maltodextrin •Fat: palm, soy, coconut, sunflower oil	•Kids with reflux •Thickens in stomach (rice starch added)
Altered electrolytes Similac® 60/40	•20 calories/ ounce •Protein: whey, casein •Carbohydrate: lactose •Fat: soy, coconut, corn oil •280 mOsm/ kg	•For kids with cardiac or renal disease •Lower calcium, phos, iron
Soy Based		
With Iron Isomil), Prosobee®, Good Start®, Supreme Soy®	•20 calories/ ounce •Protein: soy/ L- methionine •Carbohydrate: corn syrup/ sucrose (Isomil) •Fat: safflower, soy, coconut, palm, sunflower oils •200 mOsm/ kg	•Lactose intolerance •Cow's milk formula intolerance, •Galactosemia
Prosobee® 24	•24 calories/ ounce •Same as above except 240 mOsm/kg	•Same as above but ↑ calorie needs

MCT= medium chain triglyceride

INFANT NUTRITION CONTINUED

Whey hydrolysate (partial hydrolysate)		
Good Start®	•20 calories/ ounce •Carbohydrate: lactose, maltodextrin •Protein: partially hydrolyzed whey •Fats: palm, soybean, safflower and coconut oils	May help prevent allergies in high-risk infants
Casein Hydrolysates		
Shared characteristics of all 3:	•20 calories/ ounce •Protein: casein hydrolysate, L-cysteine, L-tyrosine, L-tryptophan	May be helpful during acute GI illnesses (diarrhea)
1. Pregestimil®	•Fat: MCT (55%), corn, and sunflower oils •320 mOsm/ kg	Malabsorption (also comes in 24 calories/oz)
2. Alimentum®	•Fat: MCT (33%), safflower and soy oils •370 mOsm/ kg	Problems with formulas with intact protein, malabsorption
3. Nutramigen®	•Fat: palm, soy, coconut and sunflower oils •320 mOsm/ kg	May help ↓allergies in high-risk infants
Amino Acid Neocate®	•20 calories/ ounce •Protein: simple amino acids •Fat: vegetable oils •Carbohydrate: corn syrup solids	Child with sensitivity to multiple proteins
High MCT Portagen®	•20 calories/ ounce •Protein: caseinate •Fat 85% MCT, corn oils •Carbohydrate: corn syrup/ sucrose	↓ lipase/ bile salts, fat malabsorption, chylothorax

MCT= medium chain triglycerides

ENTERAL FORMULAS FOR OLDER KIDS (all have 30 calories/ oz)

Formula Name	Protein	Fat	Carbohydrate
PediaSure®	Whey/casein	Safflower, soy, MCT	Sucrose, Maltodextrin
Kindercal®	Casein	Sunflower, corn, MCT, canola	Sucrose, Maltodextrin
Ensure®	Casein/soy	Corn oil	Sucrose, Maltodextrin
Boost®	Milk protein	Sunflower, canola, corn	Sucrose/ corn
Peptamen Jr.®	Whey hydrolysate	MCT, soy, canola	Corn starch, maltodextrin

MCT= medium chain triglycerides

NUTRITION

FEEDING PRETERM INFANTS

▶ Preterm infants should gain 20- 40 grams/ day (1-1.5 ounces)
▶ Most preterm or small-for-gestational-age infants will have catch-up growth in first 3-8 months; head circumference first, then weight, then length.

Formula type	Brand names	Use
Preterm formulas (24 cals/ oz)	Enfamil Premature Lipil®, Similac Special Care®	•Infants weighing less than 2 kg (4 lbs 6 oz) and taking less than 500 mL/ day •↑ protein, vitamins A, D, B6
Transitional formulas (22 cals/ oz)	Enfamil EnfaCare Lipil®, Similac NeoSure Advance®	•↑protein, calcium, phosphorus, vitamins and other minerals
Specialized formulas	Pregestimil®, Alimentum®, Nutramigen®, Neocate®	•Should be used for formula intolerance •Designed for term infants
Soy formula	Isomil®, ProSobee®	•Not recommended for infants <1800 g (less weight gain, growth, and albumin levels)

▶ It is generally recommended that preterm infants stay on transitional formula until 9 months corrected age, but some infants may benefit from transitional formula until 12 months corrected age. Consider on an individual basis.
▶ Solids may be started at 6 months corrected age, and cow's milk may be started at 12 months corrected age.

Indications of inadequate weight gain of premature infants/ children:

Corrected Age	Weight gain
Term- 3 months	< 20 gm/ day (< 5 oz/ wk)
3 – 6 months	< 15 gm/ day (< 3½ oz/ wk)
6 – 9 months	< 10 gm/ day (< 2 oz/ wk)
9 – 12 months	< 6 gm/ day (< 1½ oz/ wk)
1 – 2 years	< 1 kg/ 6 months (< 2 pounds/ 6 months)

Adapted from Nutrition Practice Care Guidelines for Preterm Infants In the Community, 2006; http://www.oregon.gov/DHS/ph/wic/docs/preterm.pdf

NUTRITION

MIXING INFANT FORMULA

Standard Infant Formulas: from POWDER

Caloric concentration	Amount of powdered formula (level scoop)	Water (measure first, then add powder)
20 Kcal/oz	1 scoops	60 ml (2 oz)
22 Kcal/oz	3 scoops	165 ml (5.5 oz)
24 Kcal/oz	3 scoops	150 ml (5 oz)
27 Kcal/oz	3 scoops	128 ml (4.25 oz)

Increased calorie formula from ready to use standard formula:

Caloric concentration	Amount of powder	Amount of ready to use formula (measure first)
24 Kcal/ oz	1 scoop powder	300 ml (10 oz)
27 Kcal/ oz	2 scoops powder	300 ml (10 oz)

Transitional Formulas: (EnfaCare®, NeoSure®)

Calorie concentration	Amount of powder (level scoop)	Water (measure first)
22 Kcal/ oz	1 scoop	60 ml (2 oz)
24 Kcal/ oz	3 scoops	165 ml (5.5 oz)
27 Kcal/ oz	5 scoops	240 ml (8 oz)

Human Milk Fortification: (measure breast-milk first, then add powder)

Caloric concentration	Amount of powdered human milk fortifier	Amount of breast-milk (measure first)
22 Kcal/ oz	1 packet	50 ml (1.7 oz)
24 Kcal/ oz	1 packet	25 ml (1 oz)

Adapted from Nutrition Practice Care Guidelines for Preterm Infants In the Community; 2006; http://www.oregon.gov/DHS/ph/wic/docs/preterm.pdf

NUTRITION CONTINUED

Formulas with special characteristics for older kids and adolescents

Ensure Plus®, Deliver® &Two-Cal®	•↑ calorie formulas: *Ensure Plus*®= 1.5 calories/mL •*Deliver*® and *Two-cal*®= 2 calories/mL (60 cals/ oz)
Tolerex®, Vivonex Plus®	•Amino acid formula
Peptamen Jr.®	•Hydrolyzed whey formula
Portagen®: (long term: need supplements)	•↑ concentration of MCT (86%); used in patients with ↓ lipase/ bile salts, fat malabsorption, chylothorax

MCT= medium chain triglycerides
Adapted from "Pediatric Formula Composition" pamphlet by Drs John Kerner and JoAnn Hattner, 6/99 and other sources.

▶ *Formula storage:* Discard any formula left in bottle after feeding within one hour; can keep freshly mixed formula in refrigerator for 24 hours.

▶ *Mixing formula:* Follow directions carefully. Mix with cool water. If boil first, let it cool. You do not have to warm bottle but if baby prefers it, let stand in warm water for 2-5 minutes. Test on wrist before feeding.

BREASTFEEDING

CONTENTS OF BREAST MILK

Contents of human milk are variable. Primary protein: whey; fats: variable, high in omega-3's and cholesterol; carbohydrate: lactose, oligosaccharides; calories ~ 20/oz; can add human milk fortifiers to make 24 calories/ oz for preemies

BENEFITS OF BREASTFEEDING

Benefits for baby	Benefits for mom & society
Decreased risk of allergies & asthma	↓ Postpartum bleeding
Decreased risk for many infections including diarrhea, meningitis, otitis	↓ Risk breast & ovarian cancer; possible ↓ osteoporosis
↓ SIDS & postneonatal mortality	↓ Time to prepregnancy weight
↓ Risk of type I and II diabetes	↑ Child spacing
↓ Risk certain cancers (leukemia)	↓ Health care costs
↓ Risk of obesity/ hypercholesterolemia	↓ Public health costs/special programs
↑Performance: cognitive development	↓ Environmental burden

CONTRAINDICATIONS TO BREASTFEEDING

Baby with galactosemia	Mom on chemotherapy
Mother with HTLV or HIV infection	Mom taking street/illicit drugs
Mother with untreated tuberculosis	Mom with herpes infection of breast
Mother exposed to radioactive medications/ materials	Mom on certain other drugs (see next page)

HIV=Human immunodeficiency virus, HTLV=Human T-lymphotropic virus, SIDS=Sudden infant death syndrome

BREASTFEEDING CONTINUED

SITUATIONS DURING WHICH BREASTFEEDING IS USUALLY SAFE

Hepatitis B surface antigen + or Hepatitis C +	Tobacco smoking (try to quit)
Hyperbilirubinemia	Occasional alcohol ingestion*
Cytomegalovirus +mom (past conversion), term baby	Certain medications (see below)

Wait minimum 2 hours after alcohol consumed to breast-feed.

▶ American Academy of Pediatrics (AAP) recommends exclusive breast feeding for the first 6 months of life up to 1 year (longer if desired). No pacifier until breastfeeding is well established. Baby should receive 8-12 feeds/ 24 hours in the first few weeks of life.

▶ Infant should be seen by pediatrician at 3-5 days of age and at 2-3 weeks old.

▶ Breastfed infants should get 200 IU vitamin D daily starting within 1st 2 months of life until child drinking at least 500 mL/ day vitamin D supplemented formula or milk.

▶ Breastfed infants should get 0.5-1 mg vitamin K IM after first feed (< 6 hours old).

▶ Breast milk storage: freshly expressed milk can be stored 4-6 hours at room temperature, 24 hours in cooler with ice, 5 days in refrigerator, or 3 months in freezer (2 weeks if inside refrigerator).
Pediatrics Vol. 115 No. 2 February 2005, pp. 496-506

Selected medications that are contraindicated during breastfeeding:
Bromocriptine, ergotamine, phenindione, street drugs (cocaine, phencyclidine, heroin etc.), chemotherapeutic drugs, radioisotopes, lithium

Selected medications that are secreted in breast milk that may be harmful to infant or reports of effects on infants:
Anxiolytics (*diazepam, lorazepam*, etc), antidepressants (*fluoxetine, fluvoxamine*), aspirin; caffeine; chloramphenicol, clemastine, estradiol, haloperidol, mesalamine, metoclopramide, metronidazole, nitrofurantoin, phenobarbital, phenytoin, primidone, pseudoephedrine, sulfasalazine, tinidazole

Selected medications that are generally considered safe while breastfeeding:
Acetaminophen, acyclovir, atenolol, captopril, cefazolin, ceftriaxone, clindamycin, codeine, digoxin, enalapril, folic acid, ibuprofen, isoniazid, medroxyprogesterone, methadone, naproxen, nifedipine, prednisone, rifampin, senna, spironolactone, tetracycline, tetracycline, trimethoprim/ sulfamethoxazole, valproic acid, warfarin, levonorgestrel, scopolamine

Adapted from Housestaff Manual LPCH at UCSF/ Stanford, 4th edition

NUTRITION CONTINUED

INFANT FEEDING GUIDELINES

▶ Watch for hunger cues including lip smacking, rooting, or crying.
▶ Watch baby's urine output (day 1= 1 wet diaper, day 2 = 2 wet diapers; day 3 = 3 wet diapers; > 6 days old = 6-8 diapers in 24-hour period).
▶ Watch baby's stool output (will usually change from meconium to yellow/ seedy in first 5 days).
▶ Watch baby's weight (should regain birth weight by 2 weeks and should not lose more than 10% of birth weight)

Age	Frequency	Amount
0-4 weeks	•Every 1-3 hours (timed from the beginning of the feed) •8-12 feeds/ 24 hours •Wake after 4 hours to feed	•Breastfeed 20-45+ minutes/ feed •1-3 ounces per feed if using bottle.
4-8 weeks	•Every 2-4 hours	•Breastfeed 20-45+ minutes/ feed; •2-4 ounces per feed •18-32 ounces/ day
2-6 months	•Every 2-4 hours in day •Every 6-8 hours overnight (may be 10 hrs overnight @ 6 months)	•Breastfeed 20-45+ minutes/ feed •4-6 ounces per feed •24-32 ounces/day
> 6 months	•4-5 feeds/ day, decreases as increase solid foods	•Breastfeed 20-45+ minutes/ feed •6-8 ounces/ feed (32 ounces/ day)

INTRODUCTION OF SOLID FOODS

▶ May begin solids after 4-6 months. Insufficient data to make specific recommendations about when to start which food. General guidelines:

6 months old	•Start with iron fortified cereals (4 tablespoons/ serving, 1 serving/ day).
6-9 months old	•Add pureed fruits/ veggies (4 tablespoons/ serving, 2-3 servings/ day). Avoid strawberries, citrus until older.
> 9 months old	•Meats, chicken, & small amounts of cottage cheese/ yogurt, egg yolks (3-4 servings/ day).

Resource for parents: wholesomebabyfoods.com

For infants at high risk for food allergies (family history, atopy, other allergic diseases) consider:
▶ No dairy until 12 months (milk, cheese, yogurt)
▶ No eggs until 2 years
▶ No nuts, fish/ seafood until 3 years

NUTRITIONAL REQUIREMENTS

CALORIE REQUIREMENTS

Age	Calories/ day (average)	Kcal/ kg/ Day
0-6 months	650	90-120 kcal/kg/day
6-12 months	850	
1-3 years	1200-1300	75-90 kcal/kg/day
3-7 years	1600-1800	
7-11 years	1800-2000	60-75 kcal/kg/day
11-14 years	♀2100 ♂ 2500	
15-18 years	♀2100 ♂ 3000	

PROTEIN REQUIREMENTS

Age	Grams/ day	Grams/ kg/ day
1-3 years	13	1.1
4-8 years	19	0.95
9-13 years	34	
14-18 years	♀46, ♂52	0.85

FAT REQUIREMENTS

	1-3 years	4-8 years	9-13 years	13- 18 years
Total fat (grams/day)	30-50	40-60	60-85	55-95
% of total daily calories	30-35%	25-35%		
Saturated fat	< 10% of calories in kids > 2 years			

DAILY VITAMIN/ FIBER REQUIREMENTS

	1-3 years	4-8 years	9-13 years	13- 18 years
Calcium (mg)	500	800	1300	1300
Iron (mg)	7	10	8	♀15, ♂ 11
Vitamin C (mg)	15	25	45	♀65, ♂75
Vitamin A (mg)	1000	1300	2000	♀2300, ♂3000
Fiber (grams)	~15	~20	~25	♀ 20, ♂30

Source: 1999 - 2002 Dietary Reference Intakes, Institutes of Medicine 2005 Dietary Guidelines

OBESITY

DEFINITIONS

▶ *Body Mass Index* (BMI) = wt (kg)/ ht (meters) ^{2} (see BMI tables pp. 183 & 184)
▶ Kids > 2 years: BMI > 85-95%ile at risk for overweight; BMI > 95%ile overweight
▶ Kids < 2 years: weight for height > 95%ile is overweight

CAUSES OF OBESITY

▶ <u>Primary obesity</u>: By far the most common cause (genetic predisposition + lifestyle). Kids usually have associated tall stature and no dysmorphic features.
▶ <u>Syndromic</u>: Prader-Willi (hypotonia, mental retardation); Bardet-Biedl Syndrome (mental retardation, pigmentary retinopathy, polydactyly, and renal abnormalities)
▶ <u>Endocrine</u>: Growth hormone deficiency, thyroid hormone deficiency, and cortisol excess; usually associated with *short* stature.
▶ <u>Medications-induced</u>: Glucocorticoids, valproic acid, risperidone

COMORBIDITIES

▶ Obstructive sleep apnea, orthopedic (including slipped capital femoral epiphysis), fatty liver, polycystic ovaries, metabolic syndrome, pseudotumor cerebri, psychosocial (negative self image & ↓ self esteem, depression, anxiety), increased suicide risk (adolescent females)

DIABETES SCREENING

▶ American Dietetic Association (ADA) recommends screening (fasting glucose) for overweight children at 10 years old or onset of puberty, and every 2 years if 2 of the following risk factors are present:

●Acanthosis nigricans	●Dyslipidemia or hypertension
●Family history of diabetes	●Native American, African-American,
●Polycystic ovarian syndrome	Hispanic, Pacific Islander

▶ Up to 25% of overweight teens have impaired glucose tolerance on oral glucose tolerance test (OGTT); 4% may have asymptomatic diabetes. So, OGTT may be useful adjunct to screening.

Fasting plasma glucose	Interpretation
<100 mg/dL	NORMAL
100-125mg/dL	Impaired fasting glucose
> 126 mg/dL	Provisional diagnosis of diabetes
Random glucose > 200 & symptoms of diabetes: Provisional diagnosis diabetes	

2-hour post glucose (75 gram) load	Interpretation
< 140 mg/ dL	Normal
140-199 mg/ dL	Impaired glucose tolerance
>200 mg/ dL	Provisional diagnosis of diabetes

OBESITY

METABOLIC SYNDROME

▶ No criteria defined for metabolic syndrome in pediatric population yet. Below are *proposed* criteria and are based on 90%ile for age:

1. *Waist circumference*

8 years	♂>71 cm , ♀>70.5 cm
12 years	♂>85 cm, ♀>83 cm
15 years	♂>95 cm, ♀>92 cm
17 years	♂>101.8, ♀>98 cm

2. *Triglycerides*

12–19 years	♂>135 mg/dL, ♀>170 mg/dL
16–19 years	♂>165 mg/ dL, ♀>168 mg/dL

3. *High-density lipoprotein (HDL) cholesterol*

6–8 years	♀>37 mg/dL, ♂>37 mg/ dL
9–11 years	♂>39 mg/ dL, ♀ >38 mg/ dL
12–15 years	♂>35 mg/ dL, ♀ >36 mg/ dL
16–19 years	♂>33 mg/ dL, ♀ >37 mg/ dL

4. *Systolic BP* > 95%ile for age and height and gender.
5. *Fasting plasma glucose* ≥100 mg/dL or 2-hour oral glucose tolerance value ≥ 140 mg/dL.

Adapted from Ornstein RM, *Adolesc Med Clin* Oct 2006; 17(3): 565-87

GENERAL INTERVENTIONS FOR OBESITY

▶ Regular scheduled visits to motivate, weigh, and answer questions.
▶ The whole family should be involved and should have goal of healthy lifestyle.
▶ Encourage exercise at least 1 hour per day (outside of school).
▶ Limit TV & video games to maximum of 2 hours per day (less is better).
▶ Decrease intake of fast foods, sweets, soda, juices, and limit portion sizes
▶ 1 pound of weight gain is equal to about 3500 *extra* calories. So, if patient can ↓ intake by 500 calories/day, they will lose 1 lb/week. If patient stops drinking 1 soda per day and change nothing else, they will lose about 15 pounds in a year.
▶ Metformin: May be useful in adolescents with impaired glucose tolerance and insulin resistance; recommend consultation with endocrinologist.
▶ Cholesterol lowering drugs may be indicated if lifestyle and diet modifications not effective (atorvastatin approved for kids > 10 years of age).

References: 1. US National Cholesterol Education Program Adult Treatment Panel II   2. *Adolesc Med Clin*, Oct 2006; 17(3): 565-87; 3. *J Clin Endocrinol Metab* , Jun 2006; 91(6): 2074-80

OPHTHALMOLOGY

CONDITIONS THAT WARRANT REFERRAL TO PEDIATRIC OPHTHALMOLOGIST

Routine referral (within weeks)	Expedited referral (within days- 1 week)	Urgent referral (within hours)
•Iris coloboma	•Anisocoria	•Orbital cellulitis
•Microphthalmos	•Cataract	•Dacryocystitis
•Congenital ptosis (by 3 months old)	•Dacryocele	•Corneal ulcer
•Pterygium (symptomatic)	•Facial nerve palsy/ exposure keratopathy	•Herpes simplex keratitis
•Persistent/ refractory conjunctivitis, subconjunctival hemorrhage, blepharitis	•Glaucoma	•Papilledema
	•Iritis	•Intraocular foreign body or embedded corneal body
•Epiblepharon	•Horner's syndrome/ 3rd nerve palsy	•Acute vision change
•Strabismus	•Corneal foreign body	•Chemical burn
•Aniridia	•Possible ocular infection (toxoplasmosis)	•Retinoblastoma
•Albinism	•Blindness	•Hyphema (layer of blood seen in cornea)
•Congenital torticollis (by 4 months old)	•Diplopia (monocular or binocular)	•Globe laceration
•Retinopathy of prematurity	•Nystagmus (acute onset)	•Significant trauma
•Syndrome/ disorder with ocular problems/ findings‡		•Suspected abuse
•Family history§		•Excessive floaters or curtain across vision
•Dacryostenosis (<6-12 months old)		•Lid laceration if tear in lid margin

‡ Down syndrome, fetal alcohol syndrome, juvenile rheumatoid/idiopathic arthritis, galactosemia, diabetes mellitus, neurofibromatosis

§ Genetic eye diseases that warrant early referral to pediatric ophthalmology if positive family history: Aniridia; Rieger, Axenfeld, or Peter's syndromes; infantile glaucoma or cataracts; Marfan syndrome (ectopia lentis); microphthalmia; neurofibromatosis; retinitis pigmentosa; retinoblastoma; chorioretinal coloboma; high refractive errors.

INDICATIONS FOR OPHTHALMOLOGY OR OPTOMETRY REFERRAL FOR VISUAL ACUITY

Age	Refer
<3 years	If any suspicion, significant family history or exam abnormality
3-5 years	Acuity < 20/40 or 2 line difference between eyes.
≥6 years	Acuity < 20/30 or 2 line difference between eyes.

Pediatr Clin North Am. 2003; 50(1):41-53; *Pediatrics* 2002; 110(1): 187-191

STRABISMUS

▶ Corneal light reflex test or cover test should be used to diagnose strabismus.

Non-paralytic Strabismus (normal extraocular muscles)	Esotropia (>50%) (inward deviation)	•Intermittent: Common in infants; usually ↓ by 3 months of age •Pseudostrabismus: Wide nasal bridge; outgrow •Congenital: Onset < 6 months; surgical correction •Accommodative: 2-3 years, glasses
	Exotropia (outward deviation)	•Intermittent: 6 months-4 years •Constant: Congenital, neurologic, or due to bony abnormality
Paralytic Strabismus (may ↑ with eye movement)	CN 3 palsy	•Congenital: Usually secondary to birth trauma •Acquired: Intracranial mass; inflammation
	CN 4 palsy	•Congenital or acquired (trauma): Hypertropia when look to nose; head tilt generally present
	CN 6 palsy	•Congenital (rare): Transient palsy to 6 wks •Acquired: ↑ICP, Gradenigo syndrome (see below)

CN=cranial nerve, ICP=Intracranial pressure

SYNDROMES ASSOCIATED WITH STRABISMUS

•Duane syndrome: Retraction of the globe on adduction
•Brown syndrome: Cannot elevate eye in adduction
•Gradenigo syndrome: Cranial nerve 6 palsy associated with acute otitis media
•Parinaud syndrome: Vertical gaze palsy
•Angelman, Apert, Crouzon, Fetal Hydantoin, Turner, Noonan, Prader-Willi

NYSTAGMUS

Type	Description	Possible causes
Gaze evoked	•Keeping extreme eye position	•Benign ("end point") if minor & no other anomaly
Seesaw	•↑ one eye, ↓other eye; alternating	•Midbrain/pituitary lesions
Horizontal	•Slow to normal side, jerk back	•Unilateral cerebral disease
Pendular	•Equal speed in each direction	•Brainstem/ cerebellar, demyelinating disease
Downbeat	•Idiopathic, heat stroke, Arnold-Chiari malformation, multiple sclerosis, trauma, drugs (alcohol)	
Upbeat	•Cerebellar or medullary lesions, benign paroxysmal vertigo	
Periodic alternating	•Fast phase for 1-2 minutes, rest, then opposite direction, repeat	•Posterior fossa tumors, trauma, degeneration
Spasmus nutans	•Nystagmus (small/fast), head nodding, torticollis	•Onset 3-15 months, resolves 3-6 years
Vestibular	•Peripheral: one direction; fast away from lesion; horizontal; ±tinnitus •Central: 1 or 2 directions; may be vertical/ torsional	

Adapted from Bardorf, C, Nystagmus, www.emedicine.com, accessed April 5, 2006

CONJUNCTIVITIS

Type	Exam findings	Associated symptoms	Treatment
Viral [adenovirus, herpes simplex (HSV), varicella zoster (VZV), others]	•Bilateral, conjunctival injection and chemosis •Clear discharge (may stick together in a.m.) •Pre-auricular nodes •HSV and VZV: dendrites on fluorescein exam	•Fever, cold symptoms, cough •HSV & VZV: Usually have vesicular lesions around eye/ eyelids/ nose •Vision changes •Photophobia	•Highly contagious •No specific treatment except: 1. HSV: topical antiviral (95% cure, see table next page) 2. VZV: PO acyclovir (within 72hours); •HSV & VZV: to ophthalmology
Bacterial (Staph, Strep pneumo, chlamydia, Neisseria gonorrhea)	•Unilateral or bilateral •Purulent discharge, crusting •Erythema is superficial and ↑ at periphery of eye •+/-preauricular nodes •Papillary reaction •Gonococcus: copious discharge	•Mild pain or foreign body sensation •Chlamydia and gonorrhea may be associated with genital or other infection.	•Antibiotic drops (see chart next page) •Chlamydia (adults) azithromycin 1g PO single dose •Gonorrhea (GC): ceftriaxone IM + topical drops •GC & Chlamydia: to ophthalmology
Allergic (caused by variety of aeroallergens)	•Unilateral or bilateral •Watery/ stringy discharge •Itching •Injection and swelling of lids/ palpebral conjunctiva •Cobblestoning	•Exposure to allergen •Itchy nose •Itchy throat •Rhinorrhea •Sneezing •May be isolated eye findings	•Systemic or topical treatment (see chart next page) •Refractory: Topical steroids (in consultation with ophthalmology)
Vernal (Type of allergic conjunctivitis)	•Cobblestoning •Mucous/ stringy discharge •↑ risk African Americans	•Itching eyes •Photophobia •FB sensation	•Mast cell stabilizers •Topical steroids •Possibly topical cyclosporine
Ophthalmia neonatorum	See Neonatology page 119		

Pasternak A - *Clin Fam Pract* - 2004 Mar; 6(1); 19-33

CONJUNCTIVITIS CONTINUED

DIFFERENTIAL DIAGNOSIS (in addition to above causes): Kawasaki disease, foreign body, corneal abrasion, keratitis (corneal inflammation), burn (ultraviolet light/ chemical), dry eyes, glaucoma, uveitis (redness, pain, photophobia, "floaters", vision change; can be associated with juvenile arthritis, ankylosing spondylitis, toxoplasmosis, sarcoid, inflammatory bowel disease), nasolacrimal duct obstruction

COMMON OPHTHALMIC MEDICATIONS

	Minimum age	Prescription
TOPICAL ANTIHISTAMINES		
Emedastine (Emadine)	3 years	1 gtt affected eye up to qid
MAST CELL STABILIZERS (best as preventative medication)		
Lodoxamide tromethamine (Alomide)	2 years	1-2 gtts affected eye qid
Nedocromil (Alocril)	3 years	1-2 gtts affected eye bid
TOPICAL ANTIHISTAMINES + MAST CELL STABILIZERS		
Olopatadine (Patanol)	3 years	1-2 gtts affected eye bid – qid
Ketotifen (Zaditor)	3 years	1-2 gtts affected eye bid- tid
Epinastine (Elestat)	3 years	1 gtt affected eye bid
Azelastine (Optivar)	3 years	1 gtt affected eye bid
TOPICAL NON-STEROIDAL ANTI-INFLAMMATORIES (NSAIDS)		
Ketorolac tromethamine (Acular) 0.5 %	3 years	1 gtt affected eye qid
TOPICAL ANTIBIOTICS		
Polymyxin B + trimethoprim (Polytrim)	> 2 months	1-2 gtts q 3-6 hours (max 6 gtts/ day)
Ofloxacin 0.3% (Ocuflox)	1 year	1-2 gtts q 2-4 hours x 2 days then qid x 5 days
Moxifloxacin (Vigamox)	1 year	1 gtt tid for 7 days. (0.5%)
TOPICAL ANTIVIRALS		
Vidarabine (Vira-A)	2 years	½ inch ribbon 5x daily for 5-7 days
Trifluridine eye drops	6 years	1 gtt 9 times daily x 21 days

Gtt=drops

Pasternak A - Clin Fam Pract - 2004 Mar; 6(1); 19-33

BACK PAIN (Also see table on next page)

RED FLAGS FOR SERIOUS CAUSE OF PEDIATRIC LOW BACK PAIN

•Age < 4 years old	•Limits participation in play/sports	•Recent trauma
•Visible back deformity	•Limitation of range of motion	•Shift in posture
•Duration > 4 weeks	•Abnormal neurologic finding	•Fever
•Pain at night	•Not relieved by heat or NSAIDs	

Basic back anatomy	Anterior Structures	Posterior Structures
Structures	•Vertebral body •Intervertebral disks	•Facet joints •Spinous processes •Pars interarticularis
Normal Function	•Load bearing	•Control motion of back
Mechanism of injury	•Excessive load •Any motion	•Excessive motion •Any load
Pain associated with:	•**Sitting, flexion, lifting,** cough, sneeze, straining, lying supine, twisting	•**Standing, arching, rotation,** walking, tilting, running, lying prone, walking downhill
Sports associated with damage	•Weightlifting, rowing, gymnastics, tennis	•Gymnastics, diving, soccer, volleyball, tennis, ballet
Studies for evaluation	•CT scan or MRI	•X-rays: AP, lateral and oblique

Management options based on signs & symptoms

Level	Associated signs & symptoms	Management
I	•No systemic symptoms (fever), normal exam •Occasional minor trauma	•Often no studies •Follow-up 1-2 weeks
II	•Non-specific history (though no fever) •Minor exam findings (tight hamstrings, spinal asymmetry)	•AP, lateral, oblique plain radiographs of lumbosacral spine
III	•Non-specific history •May have systemic signs (fever) •Similar exam findings to above (Level II)	•Radiographs as above •CBC, ESR •Bone scan if ↑ESR
IV	•History unclear, though often report fever •Exam findings common •+/- neurologic deficit	•All above studies •Urgent MRI or CT

Adapted with permission, Tarascon Pocket Orthopaedica 2nd Edition, Tarascon Publishing, Lompoc, CA 2007

AP=anteroposterior, CBC=complete blood count, CT=computed tomography, ESR=erythrocyte sedimentation rate, NSAID=Non-steroidal anti-inflammatory drugs, MRI=magnetic resonance imaging,

BACK PAIN – DIFFERENTIAL DIAGNOSIS

Diagnosis	History & Exam	Lab/Radiology	Treatment
Muscle strain & Overuse injury	•Repetitive exercise •Tender paraspinal	•None necessary •Normal neuro exam	•Rest, stretching, heat, non-steroidal anti-inflammatory drugs (NSAIDs)
Spondylolysis •Defect of pars interarticularis •Prevalence (5–7%)	•Repetitive flexion exercise (gymnastics, diving) •Limited flexion •Tight hamstrings	•Lumbosacral X-rays: AP, lateral, oblique •Bone scan	•Asymptomatic: Re-examine every 6 months •Pain: Immobilization (body jacket or underarm orthosis) •Surgery: Pain despite immobilization
Spondylolisthesis •Vertebral body slip from spondylolysis	•Common at L5–S1 •Limited lumbar flexion •Rare neurologic findings	•X-rays as spondylolysis •Consider MRI for neurologic signs	•Goal is treatment prior to severe slip •Painless slip <25%: Observation •Slip >25% or pain: Posterior spinal fusion
Discitis •Inflammatory loss of disk height	•Stiff, straight posture •↓ flexion lumbar spine •Occasional fever	•↑ ESR •MRI(+early):Narrow disk space, irregular end plate	•If bacterial (S. aureus) cause suggested, nafcillin, cefazolin, or vancomycin x 4–6 weeks •Aspiration by CT guidance if prolonged course
Epidural abscess	•Fever, pain, hunched over	•MRI or CT+	•Neurosurgical intervention
Ankylosing spondylitis	•↓flexion lumbar spine •Arthritis of knee or foot	•HLA-B27+, rheumatoid factor negative •↑ESR	•Naproxen +/- sulfasalazine •Range of motion exercises for spine •25% have anterior uveitis: refer ophthalmology
Disk injury	•Paraspinal or sciatic pain •Worse with sitting, flexion	•Plain films normal •MRI: bulging disk	•NSAIDs, correct posture, stretch hamstrings •Avoid stress to disk, muscle relaxants
Neoplasm: •Osteoma •Neuroblastoma	•Back pain, weakness, scoliosis, neurologic findings	•Bone scan or MRI to localize lesion	•Referral to peds oncology: combination of surgery, radiotherapy & chemotherapy

ORTHOPEDICS - LIMP

Cause of limp	Presentation	Workup/ Treatment
Toxic synovitis (peak age 2-6 years, ♂>♀)	Afebrile or low grade fevers; nontoxic; limited range of motion of involved joint; ½ follow viral infection	CBC, ESR, CRP usually normal. X-rays normal; supportive care, pain control & close follow-up
Septic arthritis (usually < 5 years old, peak < 1 year old)	Refusal to bear weight; usually febrile; ± toxic appearance; hip held flexed/ externally rotated; ± warmth/ swelling at joint	Elevated WBC count, ESR & CRP; synovial fluid analysis indicated; MEDICAL EMERGENCY
Osteomyelitis (usually < 5 years old, pelvic ~ 8 years old)	Pain, fever, ± swelling/ erythema	↑ WBC, ESR, CRP; blood culture positive in 50%; ± x-rays (may see soft tissue swelling at metaphysis early; more reliable after 7-21 days); bone scan/ MRI diagnostic; admit
Discitis (toddlers)	Refusal to walk or sit; decreased range of motion spine; ± fevers	Usually increased WBC, ESR, CRP; x-ray may show disc space narrowing; MRI diagnostic; admit
Psoas muscle abscess (variable age)	Fever, back pain, limp; may see abdominal or genitourinary pain; hip held flexed and child has pain when extended (positive "psoas sign"); may be idiopathic, hematogenous spread, or associated with pyelonephritis, Crohn's disease, appendicitis	Usually increased WBC, ESR, CRP; CT is diagnostic; usually caused by *S. aureus*; treated by surgical drainage

Predictors of Septic Hip

ESR > 40 mm/hr
WBC > 12,000/mm^3
T > 38.5° C (101.5°F)
Refusal to bear weight
CRP > 2 mg/dL

J Bone Joint Surg 2006; 88A:1254

Probability of Septic hip vs toxic synovitis based on predictors

No predictors: 16.9% chance
1 predictor: 36.7% chance
2 predictors: 62.4% chance
3 predictors: 82.6% chance
4 predictors: 93.1% chance
5 predictors: 97.5% chance

ORTHOPEDICS - LIMP CONTINUED

Cause of limp	Presentation	Workup/ treatment
Trauma/ fracture (any age, consider abuse if non-ambulatory)	History of trauma? Assess for deformity, neurovascular status, and associated injuries. Assess social situation and consider abuse especially with certain types of fractures.	Labs usually normal; x-rays typically diagnostic though consider Salter Harris I if x-rays negative but tender at epiphysis
Tumors (long bone or spine, usually > 10 years old)	Pain; ± swelling/ mass; nocturnal pain; may have systemic symptoms (fevers, lethargy, anorexia)	May see increased WBC, ESR, CRP; x-rays usually positive; possibilities include leukemia, Ewing's sarcoma, metastases, osteosarcoma, bone cysts
Developmental hip dysplasia (toddlers)	Trendelenburg gait, usually painless, leg asymmetry	X-rays or ultrasound diagnostic; Orthopedic referral
Slipped capital femoral epiphysis (8-16 years old, ♂>♀)	Obese; afebrile; hip flexed and externally rotated; Trendelenburg gait; may present with hip or knee pain; 30% bilateral	CBC, ESR, CRP negative; hip x-ray diagnostic; make non- weight bearing immediately and refer.
Neuromuscular disease (toddlers)	No pain but abnormal gait present; other neurologic exam abnormality present (tone, reflexes)	CBC, ESR, CRP normal. Other workup/ referral as indicated by exam
Legg-Calvé-Perthes disease (4-9 years old, ♂>♀)	Osteonecrosis/ avascular necrosis of femoral head; pain often referred to thigh; 20% bilateral; decreased internal rotation/ abduction hip	10% familial; labs normal; hip x-rays are diagnostic
Acute rheumatic fever	Fever, migratory arthritis (large joints), carditis, erythema marginatum, subcutaneous nodules	Increased WBC, CRP, ESR; prolonged pr internal on EKG; preceding group A strep infection
Lyme disease	Brief arthritis attacks, carditis, erythema migrans, malaise	Serologic testing, see www.cdc.gov
Spondyloarthropathies, systemic lupus erythematosus, juvenile idiopathic arthritis: please see next page		

References: Atkinson C, CMAJ , 2006; 174(7): 924; Frick SL, Orthop Clin North Am , 2006; 37(2): 133-40; Pineda C, Infect Dis Clin North Am , 2006; 20(4): 789-825; Hahn RG, Am Fam Physician , 2005; 71(10): 1949-54; DePietropaolo DL, Am Fam Physician, 2005; 72(2): 297-30

LIMP CONTINUED

JUVENILE IDIOPATHIC/ RHEUMATOID ARTHRITIS (JIA/ JRA)

	Age	Signs	Other
Pauciarticular	< 8 years old	< 4 joints swollen; usually minimal-no pain	↑ risk eye complications if onset < 6 years
Polyarticular	1-6, or 11-16 years old	≥ 5 joints involved; morning stiffness, swollen joints, but minimal-no pain	(highest risk in 1st 4 years after diagnosis); eye exam every 3-6 months
Systemic Onset	Variable	Daily spiking fever, rash, ± hepato-splenomegaly, lymphadenopathy, joint swelling/ stiffness	Low risk eye involvement: eye exam yearly

SPONDYLOARTHORPATHIES

	Symptoms	Workup	Other
Ankylosing spondylitis	♂>♀; sacroiliitis, morning stiffness, arthritis in > 1 joint	HLA-B27 positive; lumbar films may show changes	May have symptomatic uveitis
Reiter syndrome	Uveitis, arthritis, urethritis	ANA usually negative; HLA-B27 usually positive	May be postinfectious
Inflammatory bowel disease	Large joints affected	HLA- B27 usually positive, ANA usually negative	May precede gastrointestinal findings
Psoriasis	Psoriasis of skin; arthritis	HLA B27 usually positive	Arthritis may precede skin findings

HLA-B27=Human Leukocyte Antigen-B27; ANA= Anti-nuclear antibodies

SYSTEMIC LUPUS ERYTHEMATOSUS

▶ Arthritis usually symmetric, painful; adolescent ♀ most common.

▶ ± Rash, fever, adenopathy, carditis, hepatitis, cerebritis, nephritis, cytopenias

▶ Labs: + ANA (> 1:650), anti-double-stranded DNA (73%), anti-Smith (31%), anti-cardiolipin, anti-ribonucleoprotein (RNP) antiphospholipid antibodies, ↓ complement levels (C3, C4; may signal flares); CBC (may see increased WBC count, variable platelets, anemia), erythrocyte sedimentation rate (elevated)

Reference: Am Fam Physician , 2006; 74(2): 293-300

SCOLIOSIS

Types of idiopathic scoliosis

Infantile	Onset < 3 years old	♂>♀; left thoracic curve common; high rate spontaneous resolution
Juvenile	Onset 3-10 years old	♀>♂; right thoracic curve common; most progress and require treatment
Adolescent	Onset > 10 years old	♀>♂; ↓ progression risk if older (nearing spinal maturity) or small curve; ↑ risk if younger/ larger curve

► Causes of scoliosis: Idiopathic, connective tissue disease (Marfan, Ehlers-Danlos), tumors (Neurofibromatosis), neuromuscular disease (cerebral palsy, muscular dystrophy), bone anomalies (hemivertebrae).

► US Preventative Task Force recommends against the routine screening of adolescents for idiopathic scoliosis (interventions for mild scoliosis unlikely to help most patients; severe scoliosis likely to be identified without screening).

► Scoliosis is identified by "C" or "S" curve of back, unequal shoulder heights, rib "hump" with forward flexion. X-rays ("scoliosis series") to measure angle.

Management of variable degrees of scoliosis:

< 20°	• < 20° *and* skeletally immature, recheck in 3-6 months • <20° and skeletally mature, recheck in 6-12 months. Unlikely to progress
> 20° or progressing	• Consider orthopedic consultation and bracing. • Milwaukee brace or Thoracolumbosacral orthosis (TLSO) • ↑ time in brace→↑ success.
> 30°	• Orthopedic consultation.

RESOURCES: www.scoliosis-assoc.org, www.niams.nih.gov
References: *American Family Physician* 71 (10); 2005

KNEE AND ANKLE INJURIES

► Evaluate for associated injury, open wounds, neuro-vascular status. Always consider Salter-Harris I fracture if tender near physis and X-ray negative.

	Examination	Radiographs
Ankle	Consider x-rays if tender near a malleolus and difficulty bearing weight.	AP, lateral and mortise views
Knee	Anterior drawer (anterior cruciate ligament tear), posterior drawer (posterior cruciate ligament tear), Apley compression test (meniscal injury), patellar apprehension test (patellar subluxation), tender at tibial tuberosity (Osgood- Schlatter's disease)	Anteroposterior (AP), lateral, & patellar views; consider tunnel or intercondylar view

ORTHOPEDICS

Salter-Harris Classification of Physeal Injuries (*JBJS* 45A:587-622, 1963)

Type	Description	Characteristics
I	Transverse through growth plate	Younger age
II	Same as Type I with a metaphyseal fragment (Thurston-Holland fragment)	Older age (>10)
III	Through growth plate with extension through epiphysis into joint	Intra-articular
IV	Through epiphysis and metaphysis	↑ Risk of growth arrest
V	Crush injury to the growth plate	Late growth arrest
VI	Damage to the perichondral ring of LaCroix	Physeal bridge/ asymmetric growth irregularity (angular deformity)

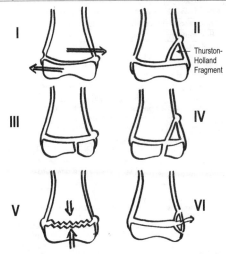

CRANIOSYNOSTOSIS/ SKULL DEFORMITIES

(looking down onto top of head)

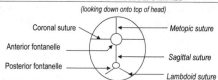

Craniosynostosis: Premature closure of suture(s) →impaired head growth and deformity [~20% associated with syndrome (Crouzon, Apert's), ~80% isolated]
Deformational Plagiocephaly: Positional molding; risk factors: multiple gestation, prematurity, forceps/vacuum delivery, excessive time in car seat, minimal "tummy time", torticollis, head position not altered when supine; affects up to 50% of infants; most often confused with lambdoid synostosis, which is very rare (incidence of 0.003%). Diagnosis of deformational plagiocephaly is made clinically.

Deformational Plagiocephaly	Lambdoid craniosynostosis
Head usually normal at birth	Usually present at birth
Parallelogram shape when looking down at top of head	Flat occiput, minimal to no frontal bossing
Side with flattened occiput has frontal bossing, prominent zygoma and anteriorly displaced ear.	Side with flattened occiput has posteriorly displaced ear. Minimal to no facial deformity.

Other forms of craniosynostosis

Scaphocephaly (sagittal synostosis): Most common form; "boat shaped" head
Turricephaly (coronal synostosis): "Tower shaped head"
Trigonocephaly (metopic synostosis): Pointed forehead

Expected times of closure for fontanelles/ sutures

Anterior fontanelle: 4-24 mos	*Early*: May be normal; check head circumference & look for head deformity (see above)
Posterior fontanelle: 2 mos	*Late*: Hypothyroidism, Down syndrome, hydrocephalus, rickets

WORKUP: (consider if diagnosis in question or if severe/ progressive deformity)
▶ *Plain radiographs* may show obliterated suture.
▶ *Head CT* more sensitive. May show premature bridging of bone across suture.
MANAGEMENT:
▶ Deformational plagiocephaly: Supervised "tummy time", minimize time in car seat, alternate head position, neck muscle stretching if torticollis present.
▶ If progression despite > 3 mos of above intervention, refer to neurosurgery to confirm diagnosis & cranial remolding orthosis (best time to treat is 4-12 mos old)
▶ If abnormal radiographs or CT, refer to neurosurgery promptly.

COMMON PEDIATRIC ORTHOPEDIC PROBLEMS

INTOEING

▶ Measure foot progression angle (long axis of foot relative to straight line in direction child is walking). Normal is 0-30° of external rotation.

▶ <u>Internal Tibial Torsion</u>: Measure thigh foot axis (child prone and knee flexed; angle bottom of foot makes relative to thigh). Normal is 0-30° external rotation. Consider referral if: asymmetric (>10°difference), severe (> 15°), or progressive after 20 months of age (consider Blount's disease).

▶ <u>Excessive Femoral Anteversion</u>: most common in girls > 3 years old. Exam shows > 70°internal hip rotation (child prone, knee flexed; measure how far can rotate leg toward exam table). >95% resolve by 8 years of age without treatment.

OUTTOEING

▶ Caused by decreased femoral anteversion, external rotation contracture of newborn hips (toddler), or external tibial torsion. Usually spontaneously resolves by 8 years.

▶ *Red flags*: progressive or asymmetric (consider developmental hip dysplasia, coxa vara, slipped capital femoral epiphysis, progressive flat foot deformity).

GENU VARUM ("bowlegs")

▶ Examine child laying down with knees extended and patella directly anterior.

▶ Red flags: Asymmetry (> 10°difference between knees) or does not follow physiologic knee changes (see table below)

▶ Non-physiologic causes include Blount's disease ("beaking" of proximal medial tibial metaphysis on x-ray), vitamin D resistant rickets, hypophosphatemia, achondroplasia, tumors, post-traumatic physeal arrest, or late onset Blount's disease.

Physiologic knee changes:

Infant up to 20 months old:	Up to 15° genu varum
2.5- 5 years old:	Up to 15° genu valgum
By 8 years of age:	5-10° genu valgum

GENU VALGUM ("knock knees")

▶ Red Flags: Progressive, asymmetric, or > 15° deformity (refer to orthopedist).

▶ Non physiologic causes include rickets, renal osteodystrophy, post -traumatic malunion or overgrowth, tumors, congenital anomalies, myelomeningocele, poliomyelitis.

BAKER'S CYST: Cystic mass palpated below popliteal fossa; rest, ice, NSAIDS.
SEVER'S DISEASE: Pain at bottom of heel; treat with cushions, rest, NSAIDS.

Assessment of Angulation And Torsion of Lower Limbs in Children, Stricker, *International Peds* Vol 16 3/ 01

ASTHMA

<u>Definition</u>: Airway hypersensitivity resulting in chronic inflammation and episodes of bronchospasm that are at least partially reversible

Epidemiology	Affects 5-8/100 kids, ↑ incidence in minority & urban kids
Symptoms	Intermittent or chronic wheeze, dyspnea, exercise intolerance, cough (including nighttime cough)
Triggers	Smoke, exercise, viral infection, animals, grasses, weather change
Signs	Hyperexpanded chest, expiratory wheeze, prolonged expiratory phase, nasal flaring, use of accessory muscles, boggy nasal mucosa, eczema
Severity	In ascending order of severity based on chest exam: Expiratory wheeze < biphasic wheeze < silent (minimal air movement)
Differential diagnosis	Congestive heart failure, cystic fibrosis, foreign body, GERD bronchiolitis, airway malacia, vascular ring, abnormal bronchus

Classification and step-wise treatment approach to asthma management

		Symptoms	PEF	Treatment
Step 1	Mild intermittent	Day: ≤2x/week Night: ≤2x/month	≥80% predicted	•β_2 agonist as needed •No daily controller meds
Step 2	Mild persistent	Day: 3-6 days/wk Night: ≤2x/month	≥80% predicted	•1st line: Low dose ICS •Alt: Cromolyn Leukotriene modifier
Step 3	Moderate persistent	Day: Daily Night: >1x/week	60-80% predicted	•Medium-dose ICS & •Long-acting β_2 agonist
Step 4	Severe persistent	Day: Continual Night: ≥4x/week	<60% predicted	•High-dose ICS & •Long-acting β_2 agonist ••+/- PO steroids

<u>Step-down therapy</u> every 2-4 months if patient's symptoms remain well-controlled.
<u>Step-up therapy</u> if symptomatic @ 4-5 weeks despite compliance with meds.

Peak Expiratory Flow (PEF) based on height (ht) in inches, flow in Liters/min:

Ht	43	45	47	49	51	53	55	57	59	61	63	65
PEF	147	173	200	227	254	280	307	334	360	387	413	440

SHORT-TERM RELIEF MEDICATIONS FOR OUTPATIENT THERAPY

•Albuterol HFA (90mcg/puff)	2 puffs every 4 hours as needed
•Albuterol nebulized	1.25 mg-5 mg nebulized as often as q4 hours
•Levalbuterol nebulized	0.31-1.25 mg/dose as much as 3 times daily
•Levalbuterol HFA (45mcg/puff)	1-2 puffs every 4-6 hours as needed
•Prednisone, prednisolone, or methylprednisolone	1-2 mg/kg/day (max 60 mg/day) for 3-10 days. Continue until symptoms resolve or PEF≥80%

GERD: Gastroesophageal reflux disease, HFA: Hydrofluoroalkane, ht: height, ICS: Inhaled corticosteroid,
PEF: Peak expiratory flow, PO=oral

ASTHMA CONTINUED

INHALED CORTICOSTEROIDS (ICS): Doses per day based on intensity of therapy

Generic drug name	Concentration	Dose
Beclomethasone MDI (*Beclovent, Vanceril* > 6 yrs old, *QVAR* > 5 yrs)	Beclovent/ Vanceril 42 or 84 mcg/puff	1-2 puffs tid-qid (42 mcg/puff) or 2 puffs bid (84 mcg/ puff)
	QVAR 40 or 80 mcg/puff	40 – 80 mcg bid
Budesonide DPI (*Pulmicort Flexhaler*, > 6 yrs old)	90 mcg/dose or 180 mcg/dose	1-2 puffs bid (180 mcg- 360 mcg bid)
Budesonide solution (nebulized, > 1 year old)	0.25 mg/2ml or 0.5 mg/2ml	0.5 mg – 1 mg single daily dose or divided bid
Flunisolide MDI (*AeroBid, Aerospan*, > 6 yrs)	250 mcg/puff	2 puffs bid
Fluticasone HFA (*Flovent*, > 4 years old)	44 mcg/puff	4-11 years: 88 mcg bid > 12 years: 88-440 mcg bid
	110 mcg/puff	
	220 mcg/puff	
Fluticasone DPI (*Flovent Diskus* > 4 years old)	50 mcg/dose	4-11 years: 50 mcg bid; > 12 years: start with 100 bid, max 500 mcg bid
	100 mcg/dose	
	250 mcg/dose	
Triamcinolone MDI (*Azmacort*, > 6 yrs old)	100 mcg/puff	200- 400 mcg bid-qid

DPI: Dry powder inhaler, HFA: Hydrofluoroalkane, MDI: Metered dose inhaler   Adapted with permission from Tarascon Pocket Pharmacopoeia, Tarascon Publishing, Lompoc, CA 2007

Concerns about inhaled corticosteroids:
• Systemic absorption can lead to adrenal suppression & resultant adrenal insufficiency if medication abruptly stopped. Growth suppression has been shown to be minimal (~1-2cm), and long-term studies show no difference in adult height.

ADJUNCTIVE LONG-TERM CONTROL MEDICATIONS (in addition to ICS)
• Long-acting β_2 agonist (salmeterol = *Serevent*, formoterol = *Foradil*): As effective (with ↓side-effects) as theophylline at ↓nighttime symptoms and exercise-induced symptoms. Use as an adjunct to ICS. *Not recommended* for monotherapy or for relief from acute exacerbations. Concern for increased mortality in one adult study prompted FDA warning
• Leukotriene receptor antagonist (montelukast = *Singulair*, zafirlukast = *Accolate*): >2 years old, controller only, use with ICS (not for monotherapy), useful in exercise-induced asthma.
• Mast cell stabilizers (cromolyn = *Intal*, nedocromil = *Tilade*): Use as adjunct for allergic or exercise-induced asthma; may help ↓dose of ICS
• Theophylline: Associated with headache, insomnia, nervousness.

Therapies Not Recommended: Mucolytics, chest percussive therapy, cough suppressant, & incentive spirometry all may trigger worsening bronchospasm.

National Asthma Education and Prevention Program. Expert panel report 2: Bethesda MD NHLBI 1997

BRONCHIOLITIS

PATHOPHYSIOLOGY: Acute, self limited, inflammatory disease of lower respiratory tract leading to obstruction of small airways from edema, mucous and cellular debris. *Air trapping* as ↑resistance during exhalation. *Atelectasis* when obstruction complete. Ventilation/perfusion (V/Q) mismatch leads to hypoxemia. *Hypercapnia* occurs only in severely affected infants with respiratory rates > 60-70 breaths/min, just prior to decompensation.

EPIDEMIOLOGY: Winter outbreaks, universal infection by 2 yrs of age, reinfection common. 11-12% of all infants develop bronchiolitis. 1-2% of infected infants are hospitalized. Accounts for 17% of infant hospitalizations & 200-500 deaths/year.

ETIOLOGY: Respiratory syncytial virus (*RSV*) >50% cases. Other viruses include parainfluenza type 3, mycoplasma, adenovirus, human metapneumovirus (hMPV)

RSV: Transmission by direct or close contact with contaminated secretions.
- Persists on countertops ~6 hours, rubber gloves ~90 minutes, hands ~30 minutes
- Incubation period: 2-8 days
- Viral shedding: Usually 3 - 8 days, though up to 3 - 4 weeks in infants

DIAGNOSIS: General symptoms: Fever (100-104ºF), malaise, copious rhinorrhea
- Lower respiratory symptoms: Wheezing (obstructive > bronchospasm), retractions, grunting, nasal flaring, tachypnea, hypoxia
- Exam varies: Migratory wheeze, rhonchi & crackles as infant mobilizes secretions.

LABS/RADIOLOGY

- *RSV nasal wash*: Not necessary to confirm diagnosis. Useful in rooming hospitalized patients together (cohorting) & disease surveillance.
- *Chest X-ray*: May be misleading as wandering atelectasis common (right upper lobe most common), often misinterpreted as lobar infiltrate. Hyperinflation, peribronchial cuffing & streaky perihilar infiltrates common.
- *Complete blood count*: Leukocytosis and bandemia common with RSV. Not sensitive or specific for presence of bacterial superinfection during bronchiolitis.
- *Chemistry panel*: Not necessary. Clinically assess hydration & PO capability.
- *Blood gas*: Use as clinically indicated to determine risk of respiratory compromise.

DIFFERNTIAL DIAGNOSIS

- Asthma: + family history, no URI symptoms, repeat episode, eosinophilia
- Cystic fibrosis: Failure to thrive, clubbing of digits
- Congestive heart failure: Grunting, muffled heart tones, murmur
- Pertussis: Staccato, paroxysmal cough with cyanosis +/- inspiratory "whoop"
- Pneumonia: Fixed crackles, deep cough, limited upper respiratory sounds
- Foreign body: Fixed exam, stridor, wheezing or crackles depending on location

URI=upper respiratory infection

ADMISSION CRITERIA: Severe dyspnea, dehydration, room air SaO$_2$ <90%, infant ≤ 28 days in first 48-72 hours of illness (↑apnea risk), poor social situation

TREATMENT of BRONCHIOLITIS	
Hydration	•Consider nasogastric feeds or intravenous fluids if breathing > 60-80/min and unable to maintain hydration.
Nasal Bulb Suction	•Before feeds, before respiratory treatments and as needed. •No controlled studies of efficacy or morbidity.
Racemic epinephrine	•Probable efficacy from ↓ in airway edema. •May also have some bronchodilation effect.
Supplemental O₂	•For persistent SaO₂ < 90%. Wean when SaO₂ > 90%.
Corticosteroids	•Not indicated. No Δ in hospitalization rate or length of stay. •Used in adenovirus bronchiolitis to ↓bronchiolitis obliterans.
Antibiotics	•Not generally indicated: Consider coexisting serious bacterial infection in infants < 2 months old with fever. •75% of OM associated with bronchiolitis is from RSV
β₂-adrenergic agonists	•~25% of patients respond to albuterol, though evidence shows little effect on clinical scores or hospital length of stay. Pre/post β₂-agonists evaluation essential. •Responders may be future asthmatics.
Ribavirin	•In vitro activity vs. RSV, but NOT recommended. Evidence fails to show a benefit (no change in mechanical ventilation rate, duration of PICU/hospital stay). Potential teratogen.
SaO₂ Monitors	•No change in outcome. ↑length of stay due to prolonged O₂ therapy. Consider spot SaO₂ checks instead.

•**No evidence of efficacy** for *antihistamines, decongestants, nasal vasoconstrictors, chest physiotherapy, cool mist, or aerosolized saline.*

RSV: respiratory syncytial virus, OM: otitis media; Cochrane Database Syst Rev 2007 Jan 24;(1):CD004881
Arch Ped Adoles Med 2004 Feb 158; 127-137; Pediatrics 2006 Oct 118;(4):1774-1793; NEJM 2007 Jul 26;357:331-9

PREVENTION

Contact isolation: Gown & glove with good hand washing and/or alcohol rub
Passive immunization: RSV-IVIG (*RespiGam*) or palivizumab (*Synagis*)
•Monthly IM injection for duration of RSV season (~ 5 injections). *Expensive.*
•Criteria for high risk infants to received passive RSV immunization:
  1. <2 years old with chronic lung disease (O₂, chronic steroids, bronchodilators, *and/or* diuretic requirement; cystic fibrosis)
  2. Ex-29-32 week premature infant <6 months old @ *start* of RSV season
  3. Ex-28 week or less premature infant during 1ˢᵗ RSV season
  4. Ex-32-35 week premature infant with 2 risk factors: Daycare, school-aged siblings, tobacco exposure, neuromuscular disease, or airway abnormalities
  5. < 2 years old with cyanotic heart disease *or* on medication for congestive heart failure.

PROGNOSIS: Most recover without sequelae.
•Apnea can occur in neonates, generally < 1 month old and in 1ˢᵗ 48ᵒ of illness.
•Case fatality < 1% (Causes: Prolonged apnea, respiratory acidosis, dehydration)
•Average duration of illness in children < 24 months is 12 days (18% ill at 3 weeks).
•40% have subsequent wheezing while < 5 years old & 10% wheeze > 5 years old.

CHRONIC COUGH (in a child <14 years old)

DEFINITION: (>14 years old, treat as adult)
- Daily cough lasting >4 weeks without evidence for a *specific* etiology.

HISTORY & EXAM FINDINGS CONCERNING for *SPECIFIC* ETIOLOGY:
- Wheeze, murmur, chest pain, dyspnea, tachypnea, failure to thrive, clubbing of digits, dyspnea on exertion, hypoxia, cyanosis, feeding problems, recurrent pneumonia, significant neurodevelopment abnormality, hemoptysis

TREATMENT: Avoid environmental allergens & tobacco smoke exposure.
- Antihistamines, anti-reflux therapy, over-the-counter medications not likely to help.

EVALUATION of NON-SPECIFIC CHRONIC COUGH

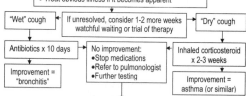

SPECIFIC CAUSES OF CHRONIC COUGH AND TESTS TO CONSIDER

Foreign body	•Bronchoscopy
Cystic fibrosis	•Sweat chloride test
Ciliary dyskinesia	•Biopsy for ciliary function studies
GERD, aspiration	•Barium swallow; pH monitoring; bronchoalveolar lavage; video swallow study
Infectious	•Chlamydia, cytomegalovirus, HIV serology, *Bordetella pertussis* culture or direct fluorescence antibody testing, tuberculosis testing, bronchoscopy, immune workup
Congenital anomaly	•Computed tomography scan; bronchoscopy; angiography; magnetic resonance imaging
Asthma	•Pulmonologist consult; pulmonary function tests
Interstitial lung disease	•Autoimmune workup •Lung biopsy
Cardiac	•Echocardiogram; electrocardiogram; catheterization

GERD: Gastroesophageal reflux disease, HIV: Human immunodeficiency virus

Chest. 2006 Jan;129: 260S-283S.

PNEUMONIA (PNA)

- Determine severity of illness based on:
  - History (age, duration of symptoms, fever, immunization status, season)
  - Physical exam (tachypnea, grunting, flaring, retractions, O_2 saturation, fever)
- Tachypnea (respiratory rate >50/min in older child) sensitive, but not specific, for bacterial pneumonia.
- Consider chest X-ray if fever without source and elevated white blood cell count.
- Follow-up X-rays only in complicated cases; may take up to 2 months to clear.
- Pneumonia, especially lower lobe, may present with abdominal pain.

PATHOGENS

Neonate	• Group B streptococcus, *Escherichia coli*, *Streptococcus pneumoniae*, Herpes simplex virus, cytomegalovirus, *Ureaplasma urealyticum*
1-4 months	• *Strep pneumo*, *Chlamydia trachomatis*, viruses, *Staphylococcus aureus*, *Moraxella catarrhalis*, *Haemophilus influenza* (Hib), *Bordatella pertussis*, *Ureaplasma urealyticum*
4 mos-4 yrs	• Viruses (respiratory syncytial virus, influenza, adenovirus), *Strep pneumo*, *Moraxella catarrhalis*, *Mycoplasma pneumoniae*, rarely Hib
≥4 years	• *Mycoplasma* or *Chlamydia pneumoniae*, *Strep pneumo*, *S aureus*, influenza

OUTPATIENT MANAGEMENT OF UNCOMPLICATED PNEUMONIA

(Admit to hospital in complicated cases, respiratory distress, dehydration, vomiting.)

Age	Management options
Neonate	• Admit for IV antibiotics (ampicillin and cefotaxime)
1-6 months	• Amoxicillin 80-100 mg/kg/day divided bid x 7-10 days, or • Erythromycin if suspect pertussis or chlamydia pneumonia
6 mos-4 yrs	• Amoxicillin 80-100 mg/kg/day divided bid-qid, or • Azithromycin 10 mg/kg day 1 (max 500 mg), then 5 mg/kg day 2-5 (max 250 mg/day)
≥4 years	• Azithromycin 10 mg/kg day 1, then 5 mg/kg day 2-5 • If > 8 years old, consider doxycycline 4 mg/kg/day divided bid

N Engl J Med 2002;346:429-437

- Chest physiotherapy (CPT), postural drainage, and mucolytics are not indicated.
- Cough may persist for >6 weeks after viral pneumonia or pertussis.

UNUSUAL CIRCUMSTANCES

Aspiration PNA	• Amoxicillin/clavulanate or penicillin G if treatment indicated
Granuloma on X-ray	• Tuberculosis, coccidiomycosis (US southwest), histoplasmosis or blastomycosis (US Midwest/Mississippi valley), sarcoidosis
Cystic fibrosis	• *Staph aureus* (<6 years old), *Pseudomonas aeruginosa* (mucoid), *Aspergillus fumigatus*, *Burkholderia cepacia*
Sickle cell anemia	• Acute chest syndrome
Bird exposure	• *Chlamydia psittaci*

OBSTRUCTIVE SLEEP APNEA SYNDROME (OSAS)

DEFINITION: Airway obstruction (partial or complete) during sleep leads to disrupted ventilation, carbon dioxide retention, and hypoxia. Screen at routine health visits by asking about snoring, disrupted sleep, daytime somnolence.

Epidemiology	Risk Factors	Symptoms
•Up to 10% preschool children snore nightly •As many as 2% have OSAS	•Obesity •Enlarged tonsils •Craniofacial anomalies •Neuromuscular disease	•Nightly snoring •Disturbed sleep •Daytime somnolence •School problems

Possible Exam Findings	Morbidity If Untreated
•Patients frequently obese •Systemic hypertension •Loud S2 (pulmonary hypertension) •Tonsillar hypertrophy	•Poor school performance •Failure to thrive •Cor pulmonale •Mental retardation

EVALUATION

- **Polysomnography (PS):** Formal sleep test that monitors sleep stage, cardiac electrical activity, respiratory rate, air flow at mouth and nares, oxygen saturation, and muscle activity. Performed in specialized centers as an overnight test. Differentiates snoring from obstructive sleep apnea.
- **Echocardiography:** Look for evidence of right ventricular hypertrophy.

TREATMENT

▶ **Adenotonsillectomy (T&A):** 1st line treatment for most children.
- Post-operative *inpatient* monitoring for T&A patients with high-risk conditions: Macroglossia, hypotonia, trisomy 21 (Down), neuromuscular disease, craniofacial anomalies, prematurity, obesity, age < 3 years old, right heart failure

▶ *If symptoms persist post-T&A*, repeat polysomnography in 6-8 weeks.
- Non-responders to T&A with abnormal polysomnography may benefit from continuous positive airway pressure (CPAP), other surgical intervention (uvulopharyngopalatoplasty), or *rarely* tracheostomy.

- Avoid sedative medications.
- Encourage weight loss.
- Treat allergic symptoms.
- Oxygen is rarely indicated (use only with continuous P_{CO_2} monitor).

Clinical practice guideline: Diagnosis and management of childhood obstructive sleep apnea syndrome.
Pediatrics 2002 Apr;109(4):704-712.

CROUP

Presentation: Ages 3-36 months (spasmodic croup may present in older children). Usually fall/ winter. Preceding upper respiratory infection, then barking cough ±inspiratory stridor. Symptoms ↑ at night; may or may not have fever.

Diagnosis: Generally clinical. X-rays may or may not show characteristic "steeple sign" (subglottic narrowing, 50% false negative rate).

Etiology: Parainfluenza 1, 2, & 3 account for 80% of cases. Influenza A causes severe disease. Also Influenza B, respiratory syncytial virus, adenovirus, metapneumovirus, enteroviruses and rarely *Mycoplasma* can cause croup.

Differential Diagnosis: Foreign body (no upper respiratory symptoms; afebrile; acute onset), epiglottitis (toxic, fever, drooling), bacterial tracheitis (toxic appearance, may be complication of croup), retropharyngeal abscess/ paratonsillar abscess, anaphylaxis.

Assessment/ Westley Croup Score[5]:

		0	1	2	3	4	5
Awareness		-	-	-	-	-	Disoriented
Cyanosis	NORMAL	-	-	-	With crying	At rest	
Stridor		With crying	At rest	-	-	-	
Air entry		↓	Marked ↓	-	-	-	
Retractions		mild	moderate	severe	-	-	

Add above points to get croup score. ≤2: mild   3-7: moderate   ≥8: severe

TREATMENT: consider hospital admission if stridor at rest, toxic, unsure diagnosis, dehydrated, unreliable followup.

Mild Croup (<2)	Moderate (3-7)	Severe (>8)	NOTES
•Avoid agitation •Dexamethasone 0.15-0.6 mg/kg PO# x 1 may ↓parental anxiety, return visits, *and* ↓severity. Child may sleep more.[2]	•Avoid agitation •Dexamethasone 0.6 mg/kg IM, IV or PO† •Nebulized epinephrine* •Consider admission	•Avoid agitation •Dexamethasone 0.6 mg/kg IM, IV or PO† •Nebulized epinephrine* •Consider ICU admission	•ABC's •Cool mist has been found anecdotally helpful, but unlikely to help in moderate to severe cases.

ABC's: Airway, breathing, circulation [basic life support (BLS) principles]

Mix IV Decadron solution (4 mg/mL) with maple syrup for PO dosing.

* Racemic epinephrine 0.05 mL/ kg / dose (max 0.5 mL) of 2.25% solution mixed with normal saline to make 3 mL, nebulized over 10-15 min; may use standard epinephrine solution 1:1000, 0.25 mL in 2.5 mL normal saline by nebulizer. Observe for 3-4 hours after administration.

†PO and IM Decadron appear to be equally effective. Maximum dose is 10 mg. Inhaled budesonide may be as effective as PO dexamethasone, but less effective than IM dexamethasone[3]. Oral prednisolone less effective than dexamethasone.[4]

1) JAMA 1998;(279):1629-32.   2) Journal of Pediatrics 2005;146(3).   3) N Engl J Med 1998;339:498-503.
4) Arch Dis Child 2006;91(7): 580-3.   5) Am. J. Respir. Crit. Care Med,1998;157(1),331-334 (croup score)

TESTICULAR PROBLEMS

Diagnosis	Onset / Symptoms	Exam / Work-up	Treatment	Outcome
Testicular torsion	Newborn or 12- 18 years; Acute onset scrotal pain; +/- history of trauma; 25% with abdominal pain; +/- nausea, vomiting, fever.	High riding testicle; very tender; ±edema; ± red; ↓cremasteric reflex; no relief with elevation; Doppler US 86% sensitive (very specific)	Urology consultation for manual detorsion (success 30-70%) or surgical detorsion/ orchiopexy	80-100% success rate if treated by 6 hours; ↓to near 0% success at 12 hrs after onset of pain.
Torsion of appendix testis	Preadolescent; slower onset; less severe than testicular torsion. No vomiting, abdominal pain.	Localized tenderness at upper testis; "blue dot" on anterosuperior scrotal wall; US shows normal/ ↑ flow.	Analgesics, scrotal support; surgery for severe pain	Excellent. No long-term morbidity.
Testicular cancer	Slow onset of painless mass/swelling; ±systemic symptoms	US, CXR, abdominal/ pelvic/ head CT for staging; hCG, alpha- fetoprotein, LDH	Radical orchiectomy; offer sperm banking	Depends on type of cancer & presence/ extent of metastases
Epididymitis / epididymo- orchitis	Scrotal pain, dysuria, urgency, frequency, swelling, abdominal pain, tender at epididymis, ↓ pain with scrotal elevation	Urinalysis (1/2 have pyuria; bacteria) & culture; DNA probe for gonorrhea/ chlamydia. Prepubertal: consider urology consult	Analgesics; elevation of scrotum; antibiotics (for positive urine culture or DNA probe)	Depends on cause: urine reflux, infection, postinfectious/ inflammatory, sexually transmitted infection
Hydrocele	Transilluminating edema, nontender, normal color	Older kids: May be caused by infection or malignancy	Surgical correction if unresolved by 1-2 years	Good prognosis (unless underlying pathology)
Varicocele	Painless, asymptomatic	"Bag of worms", ↑ size with standing	Repair if asymmetric testicular size, abnormal semen analysis, or pain	Red flags: Sudden onset, on right only, no ↓size when supine
Undescended testicles	Absent at birth, may drop by 6 months of age	Refer to urologist if still undescended @ 6 months	Treatment: hCG injections vs surgical	↑Risk of infertility, testicle cancer, torsion

URINARY TRACT INFECTION (UTI) & VESICOURETERAL REFLUX (VUR)

Epidemiology: UTI more common in ♀, uncircumcised ♂, any ♂ <1 year old, Caucasians, patients with dysfunctional voiding, vesicoureteral reflux, obstruction, family history of UTI, indwelling catheter, and/or recent sexual intercourse.

Pathogens: *Escherichia coli* (80%), *Klebsiella*, *Proteus*, *Enterococcus*. Resistance to amoxicillin & ampicillin widespread. Know local resistance patterns of E. coli to determine optimal presumptive outpatient therapy. Recent antibiotics, long-term prophylaxis, and complicated anatomy ↑risk of non-E. coli & resistant pathogen.

URINALYSIS (UA)

Nitrites	•High specificity for Gram negative rods. Low sensitivity: Gram+ bugs (enterococcus) & frequent urination (infants)
Leukocyte esterase	•Breakdown product of WBC = indirect evidence of UTI
Microscopy	•Suspicious if >8 WBC/hpf or large amount of bacteria

CULTURE: # bacteria indicative of true urine pathogen by collection method

Clean catch (single pathogen)	Catheterization	Suprapubic aspiration
>100,000 CFU/ml	>10-50,000 CFU/ml	>1000 CFU/ml

CFU: Colony forming units, hpf: high-powered field, WBC: White blood cell

Treatment of acute UTI patient based on age at presentation:

<30 days	•IV ampicillin + either gentamicin or cefotaxime X 10-14 days (entire course is given IV given possible hematogenous origin of UTI)
30 days– 2 mos	•IV cefotaxime, gentamicin, and cefepime until afebrile, no emesis, culture and sensitivity (C&S) known; then PO to complete 7-14 days
2 mos – 2 years	•Non-toxic, no emesis: Amoxicillin/ clavulanate (AM/CL), trimethoprim/ sulfamethoxazole (TMP/SMX), or cefixime PO x 7-14 days. •Toxic or vomiting: IV ceftriaxone or gentamicin initially. Switch to PO when afebrile, no emesis, C&S known. Complete 10-14 day course
>2 years	•Trimethoprim/sulfamethoxazole, amoxicillin/clavulanate PO x 3-5 d

IMAGING: No consensus, but multiple expert-panel guidelines exist.

•Renal ultrasound (US): Identifies structural abnormalities: Hydronephrosis, perinephric abscess, calculi. Indicated if no prenatal US, poor follow-up, abnormal voiding pattern, abdominal mass, or symptoms >48-72 hours despite antibiotics.

•Contrast voiding cystourethrogram (VCUG): Most sensitive test for VUR. Large radiation dose to pelvis. Perform *after* urine infection resolved *and* voiding normal (often within 3 days of treatment). See screening recommendation next page.

•Radionucleotide cystography (RNC): Used for follow-up of known VUR. RNC=1/100th radiation of VCUG, but ↓sensitivity & less accurate at grading reflux.

•DMSA (99mTc Dimercaptosuccinic acid) scan: Sensitive for renal scars; only necessary if will change management.

•Complicated UTI: Indwelling catheter, structural anomalies (reconstructed bladder), or functional defect (neurogenic bladder) leading to difficult to clear infection and/or unusual pathogens.

•*Ciprofloxacin* FDA approved for complicated UTI in patients >1 year old

VESICOURETERAL REFLUX (VUR)

▶ **Epidemiology:** 30-40% young children with febrile urinary tract infection (UTI) and ~1% all newborns have VUR. May predispose to recurrent infection, renal scarring, hypertension, glomerular dysfunction and end-stage renal disease.

▶ **Screening Recommendations**

Male, any age	VCUG after 1st UTI (febrile or afebrile)
Female < 3 yrs old	VCUG or RNC after 1st UTI (febrile or afebrile)
Female 3-7 yrs old	VCUG or RNC after 1st febrile UTI or recurrent afebrile UTI
Female ≥ 7 yrs old	VCUG or RNC for recurrent UTI

Familial concurrence of VUR ~25%: Consider RNC for siblings <6 years old.
RNC: Radionucleotide cystogram, VCUG: Voiding cystourethrogram   N Engl J Med, 2003; 348(3): 195-202.

- **Grade I:** Reflux of urine into ureter; no dilation of ureter
- **Grade II:** Reflux into ureter & renal pelvis without dilation
- **Grade III:** Mildly dilated ureter, collecting system and blunting of calyces
- **Grade IV:** Grossly dilated ureter & collecting system. Half of calyces blunted.
- **Grade V:** Tortuously dilated ureter, all calyces blunted, possible cortical thinning

▶ **Management of VUR (by grade):** Resolution in 1st 5 yrs of life common. Depends on age, laterality, and grade of VUR. Resolution calculator @ deflux.com

| Grade I-III | • Antibiotic prophylaxis still standard of care, though controversial.
• Repeat VCUG or RNC in 6-18 months.
• If >6 years old with bilateral VUR or scarring, refer to urologist. |
| Grade IV-V | • Antibiotic prophylaxis & refer to urologist for evaluation.
• <2 yrs old, often watch & wait with repeat VCUG/RNC every 6-12 mos.
• >2 yrs, failed prophylaxis, poor visual situation or high-grade renal scarring, consider reimplantation vs. endoscopic peri-ureteral hyaluronidase injection. |

▶ **PROPHYLAXIS:** Current standard of care for recurrent UTI, renal scarring, VUR (until resolution), or obstruction. Controversial as to whether prevents scarring.

| <2 months old | Cephalexin 2-3 mg/kg PO once daily |
| >2 months old | TMP/SMX 2 mg TMP/kg po or nitrofurantoin 1-2 mg/kg po daily |

- **Goal of treatment** is *prevention of renal scarring*: Theoretically possible by changing risk factors (recurrent UTI, delay in treatment, VUR, urologic obstruction).
- **Surveillance** (when not ill) may present with recurrent UTI, test of cure urine cultures not necessary.
- **Dysfunctional voiding:** May present with recurrent UTI, urge incontinence, or abnormal voiding pattern. Comorbid constipation common. Treatment: Scheduled voids, constipation management, urology consultation, possibly anticholinergics.

PRENATAL HYDRONEPHROSIS: Consider prophylaxis while awaiting studies:

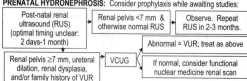

CONVERSIONS

LIQUID MEASURE:
1 teaspoon = 5 mL
1 tablespoon = 15 mL

LENGTH:
inches = 0.39 x cm
cm = 2.54 x inches

WEIGHT:
1 pound = 0.45359 kg
1 kg = 2.2 pounds
Ideal Body Weight (kg) = height $(cm)^2$ x 1.65/ 1000 (kids 1-18 years)
Body Mass Index= BMI = weight (kg)/ height $(m)^2$

TEMPERATURE:
$°F = (°C \times 9/5) + 32$
$°C = (°F-32) \times 5/9$

BODY SURFACE AREA:
BSA $(m^2) = \sqrt{[\text{height (cm)} \times \text{weight (kg)}/ 3600]}$

ESTIMATED CREATININE CLEARANCE = K x length (cm)/ serum creatinine
●K Values

< 1 year low birthweight infant: K = 0.33		< 1 year normal infant: K = 0.45	
2-12 yrs (♀ or ♂): K = 0.55	♀ 13-21 years: K = 0.55		♂ 13-21 years: K= 0.70

GROWTH RULES OF THUMB:
●Birth weight regained by 2 weeks; doubles by 4 months; triples by 1 year;
   quadruples by 2 years.
●Head circumference increases by 1 cm/ month for the first year, 3 cm/ month in
   the second year.
●Length doubles by 4 years and triples by 13 years.

AGE NORMALS

Age	Weight (Kg)	Heart rate (beats/ minute)	Respiratory rate (breaths/ minute)
< 6 hours	2.5-5 kg	80-170	40-80
0-3 months	3-7 kg	90-170	30-55
3-6 months	5-8 kg	90-165	30-55
6-12 months	6-10 kg	80-125	30-55
1-2 years	9-13 kg	80-125	25-45
2-4 years	12-16 kg	70-115	20-35
4-6 years	15-20 kg	65-115	20-30
6-12 years	20-40 kg	60-115	18-30
> 12 years	> 40 kg	60-90	12-18

ANTIPYRETIC DOSING

ACETAMINOPHEN DOSING

Weight (pounds)	Weight (kg)	Dose (mg)	Infant drops (80mg/ 0.8 mL)	Children's elixir (160mg/5 mL)
6-11	2.7-5.3	40 mg	½ dropper	
12-17.5	5.4-7.9	80 mg	1 dropper	½ teaspoon
17.6-23	8-10.6	120 mg	1 ½ droppers	¾ teaspoon
23.5-35	10.7-16	160 mg	2 droppers	1 teaspoon
35.5-47	16.1-21.5	240 mg	3 droppers	1 ½ teaspoons
47.5-59	21.6-26.9	320 mg	4 droppers	2 teaspoons
59.5-71	27-32.3	400 mg		2 ½ teaspoons
71.5-95	32.4-43.1	480 mg		3 teaspoons

Rectal suppository:
- 80 mg, 160 mg, 325 mg or 650 mg

Chewable tablets:
- *Children's Tylenol*® 80 mg
- *Junior Strength Tylenol*® 160 mg

IBUPROFEN DOSING

Weight (pounds)	Weight (kg)	Dose (mg)	Infant drops (50mg/ 1.25 mL)	Children's elixir (100 mg/ 5 mL)
11.5-16	5.2-7.4	50 mg	1 dropper	½ teaspoon
16.5-21	7.5-9.9	75 mg	1 ½ droppers	¾ teaspoon
22-27	10-12.4	100 mg	2 droppers	1 teaspoon
27.5-32.5	12.5-14.9	125 mg	2 ½ droppers	1 ¼ teaspoons
33-43	15-19.9	150 mg	3 droppers	1 ½ teaspoons
44-65	20-29.8	200 mg		2 teaspoons
66-87	29.9-39.9	300 mg		3 teaspoons
> 88	40	400 mg		4 teaspoons

Chewable tablets:
- *Children's Motrin*® or *Advil*®: 50 mg
- *Junior Advil*® or *Motrin*®: 100 mg

BMI ESTIMATE TABLE (using inches and pounds)
BMI rounded to nearest whole number

BMI→ Height (in)↓	18	19	20	21	22	23	24	25	26	27	28	29
34	29	31	32	34	36	37	39	41	42	44	46	47
35	31	33	34	36	38	40	41	43	45	47	48	50
36	33	35	36	38	40	42	44	46	47	49	51	53
37	35	37	38	40	42	44	46	48	50	52	54	56
38	36	39	41	43	45	47	49	51	53	55	57	59
39	38	41	43	45	47	49	51	54	56	58	60	62
40	40	43	45	47	50	52	54	56	59	61	63	66
41	43	45	47	50	52	54	57	59	62	64	66	69
42	45	47	50	52	55	57	60	62	65	67	70	72
43	47	49	52	55	57	60	63	65	68	71	73	76
44	49	52	55	57	60	63	66	68	71	74	77	79
45	51	54	57	60	63	66	69	72	74	77	80	83
46	54	57	60	63	66	69	72	75	78	81	84	87
47	56	59	62	65	69	72	75	78	81	84	87	91
48	58	62	65	68	72	75	78	81	85	88	91	95
49	61	64	68	71	75	78	81	85	88	92	95	99
50	64	67	71	74	78	81	85	88	92	96	99	103
51	66	70	73	77	81	85	88	92	96	99	103	107
52	69	73	76	80	84	88	92	96	100	103	107	111
53	71	75	79	83	87	91	95	99	103	107	111	115
54	74	78	82	87	91	95	99	103	107	111	116	120
55	77	81	86	90	94	98	103	107	111	116	120	124
56	80	84	89	93	98	102	107	111	115	120	124	129
57	83	87	92	97	101	106	110	115	120	124	129	134
58	86	90	95	100	105	110	114	119	124	129	133	138
59	89	94	99	103	108	113	118	123	128	133	138	143
60	92	97	102	107	112	117	122	128	133	138	143	148
61	95	100	105	110	116	121	127	132	137	142	148	153
62	98	103	109	114	120	125	131	136	142	147	153	158
63	101	107	112	118	124	129	135	141	146	152	158	163
64	104	110	116	122	128	134	139	145	151	157	163	168
65	108	114	120	126	132	138	144	150	156	162	168	174
66	111	117	123	130	136	142	148	154	161	167	173	179
67	114	121	127	134	140	146	153	159	166	172	178	185
68	118	124	131	138	144	151	157	164	171	177	184	190
69	121	128	135	142	148	155	162	169	176	182	189	196

Weight (lbs)

BMI TABLE (using centimeters and kilograms)
BMI rounded to nearest whole number

BMI→	19	20	21	22	23	24	25	26	27	28	29
Height (cm) ↓											
88	15	15.5	16	17	18	19	19	20	21	22	23
90	15	16	17	18	19	20	21	22	22	23	24
92	16	17	18	19	20	20	21	22	23	24	25
94	17	18	19	19	20	21	22	23	24	25	26
96	17	18	19	20	21	22	23	24	24	25	26
98	18	19	20	21	22	23	24	25	26	27	29
100	19	20	21	22	23	24	25	26	27	28	29
102	19	20	21	22	23	24	26	27	28	29	30
104	20	22	23	24	25	26	27	28	29	30	31
108	22	23	24	25	26	27	29	30	31	32	33
111	23	24	25	27	28	29	30	32	33	34	35
114	24	25	27	28	29	31	32	33	35	36	37
117	26	27	28	30	31	32	34	35	36	38	39
120	27	28	30	31	33	34	36	37	38	40	41
123	28	30	31	33	34	36	37	39	40	42	43
126	30	31	33	34	36	38	39	41	42	44	46
129	31	33	34	36	38	39	41	43	44	46	48
132	33	34	36	38	40	41	43	45	47	48	50
135	34	36	38	40	41	43	45	47	49	51	52
138	36	38	39	41	43	45	47	49	51	53	55
141	37	39	41	43	45	47	49	51	53	55	57
144	39	41	43	45	47	49	51	53	55	58	60
147	41	43	45	47	49	51	54	56	58	60	62
150	42	45	47	49	51	54	56	58	60	63	65
153	44	46	49	51	53	56	58	60	63	65	67
156	46	48	51	53	55	58	60	63	65	68	70
159	48	50	53	55	58	60	63	65	68	70	73
162	49	52	55	57	60	62	65	68	70	73	76
165	51	54	57	59	62	65	68	70	73	76	78
168	53	56	59	62	64	67	70	73	76	79	81
171	55	58	61	64	67	70	73	76	78	81	84
174	57	60	63	66	69	72	75	78	81	84	87
177	59	62	65	68	72	75	78	81	84	87	90

Weight (kg)

Conversion table for lbs to kg

lb \ oz	15	14	13	12	11	10	9	8	7	6	5	4	3	2	1	0
3	1.79	1.76	1.73	1.70	1.67	1.64	1.62	1.59	1.56	1.53	1.50	1.47	1.45	1.42	1.39	1.36
4	2.24	2.21	2.18	2.16	2.13	2.10	2.07	2.04	2.01	1.98	1.96	1.92	1.90	1.87	1.84	1.81
5	2.69	2.67	2.64	2.61	2.58	2.55	2.52	2.50	2.47	2.44	2.41	2.38	2.35	2.33	2.30	2.27
6	3.15	3.12	3.09	3.06	3.03	3.01	2.98	2.95	2.92	2.89	2.86	2.84	2.81	2.78	2.75	2.72
7	3.60	3.57	3.54	3.52	3.49	3.46	3.43	3.40	3.37	3.35	3.32	3.29	3.26	3.23	3.20	3.18
8	4.05	4.03	4.00	3.97	3.94	3.91	3.88	3.86	3.83	3.80	3.77	3.74	3.71	3.69	3.66	3.63
9	4.51	4.48	4.45	4.42	4.39	4.37	4.34	4.31	4.28	4.25	4.22	4.20	4.17	4.14	4.11	4.08
10	4.96	4.93	4.90	4.88	4.85	4.82	4.79	4.76	4.73	4.71	4.68	4.65	4.62	4.59	4.56	4.54
11	5.42	5.39	5.36	5.33	5.30	5.27	5.25	5.22	5.19	5.16	5.13	5.10	5.08	5.05	5.02	4.99
12	5.87	5.84	5.81	5.78	5.76	5.73	5.70	5.67	5.64	5.61	5.59	5.56	5.53	5.50	5.47	5.44
13	6.32	6.29	6.27	6.24	6.21	6.18	6.15	6.12	6.10	6.07	6.04	6.01	5.98	5.95	5.93	5.90
14	6.78	6.75	6.72	6.69	6.66	6.63	6.61	6.58	6.55	6.52	6.49	6.46	6.44	6.41	6.38	6.35
15	7.23	7.20	7.17	7.14	7.12	7.09	7.06	7.03	7.00	6.97	6.95	6.92	6.89	6.86	6.83	6.80
16	7.68	7.65	7.63	7.60	7.57	7.54	7.51	7.48	7.46	7.43	7.40	7.37	7.34	7.31	7.29	7.26
17	8.14	8.11	8.08	8.05	8.02	8.00	7.97	7.94	7.91	7.88	7.85	7.82	7.80	7.77	7.74	7.71

Converting feet & inches to centimeters

feet \ inches	0	1	2	3	4	5	6	7	8	9	10	11
1	30.5	33	35.5	38	40.5	43	45.5	48	51	53.5	56	58.5
2	61	63.5	66	68.5	71	73.5	76	78.5	81	84	86.5	89
3	91.5	94	96.5	99	101.5	104	106.5	109	112	114.5	117	119.5
4	122	124.5	127	129.5	132	134.5	137	140	142	145	147.5	150
5	152.5	155	157.5	160	162.5	165	167.5	170	172.5	175.5	178	180.5
6	183	185.5	188	190.5	193	195.5	198	200.5	203	205.5	208.5	211

Boys: Birth to 36 Months
Length-For-Age & Weight-For-Age Percentiles

Reprinted from Centers for Disease Control and Prevention website, www.cdc.gov

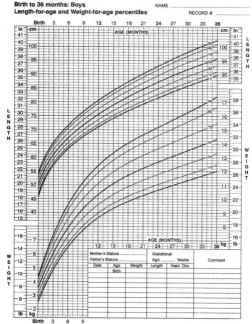

Birth to 36 months: Boys
Length-for-age and Weight-for-age percentiles

Published May 30, 2000 (modified 4/20/01).
SOURCE: Developed by the National Center for Health Statistics in collaboration with
the National Center for Chronic Disease Prevention and Health Promotion (2000).
http://www.cdc.gov/growthcharts

Boys Birth to 36 Months
Head Circumference-For-Age & Weight-For-Length Percentiles

Reprinted from the Centers for Disease Control & Prevention website, www.cdc.gov

Birth to 36 months: Boys
Head circumference-for-age and
Weight-for-length percentiles

NAME _____

RECORD # _____

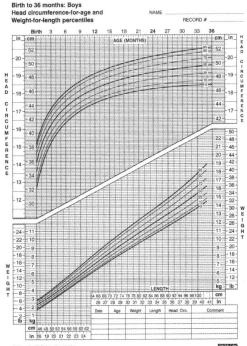

Published May 30, 2000 (modified 10/16/00).
SOURCE: Developed by the National Center for Health Statistics in collaboration with
the National Center for Chronic Disease Prevention and Health Promotion (2000).
http://www.cdc.gov/growthcharts

SAFER · HEALTHIER · PEOPLE™

Girls: Birth to 36 Months
Length-For-Age & Weight-For-Age Percentiles

Reprinted from the Centers for Disease Control & Prevention website, www.cdc.gov

---

Birth to 36 months: Girls
Length-for-age and Weight-for-age percentiles

NAME ....

RECORD # ....

		Gestational		
Mother's Stature		Age:	Weeks	
Father's Stature				Comment
Date	Age	Weight	Length	Head Circ.
	Birth			

Published May 30, 2000 (modified 4/20/01).
SOURCE: Developed by the National Center for Health Statistics in collaboration with
the National Center for Chronic Disease Prevention and Health Promotion (2000).
http://www.cdc.gov/growthcharts

SAFER·HEALTHIER·PEOPLE™

**Girls: Birth to 36 Months
Head Circumference-For-Age & Weight-For-Length Percentiles**

Reprinted from the Centers for Disease Control & Prevention website, www.cdc.gov

Birth to 36 months: Girls
Head circumference-for-age and
Weight-for-length percentiles

NAME

RECORD #

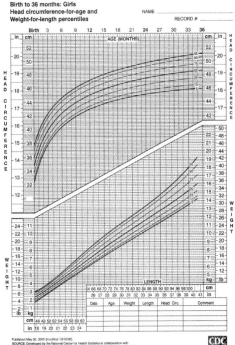

Published May 30, 2000 (modified 10/16/00).
SOURCE: Developed by the National Center for Health Statistics in collaboration with
the National Center for Chronic Disease Prevention and Health Promotion (2000).
http://www.cdc.gov/growthcharts

SAFER · HEALTHIER · PEOPLE™

Boys: 2-20 Years
Stature-For-Age & Weight-For-Age Percentiles

Reprinted from Centers for Disease Control and Prevention website, www.cdc.gov

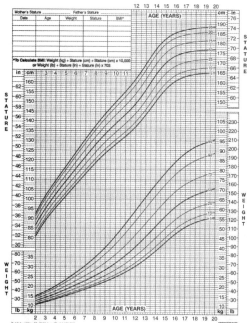

Boys: 2-20 Years
Body Mass Index-For-Age Percentiles

Reprinted from Centers for Disease Control and Prevention website, www.cdc.gov

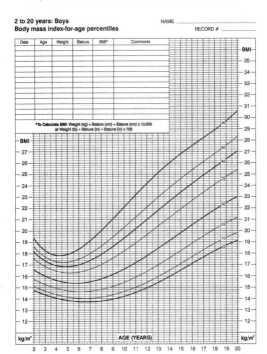

2 to 20 years: Boys
Body mass index-for-age percentiles

NAME ....

RECORD # ....

*To Calculate BMI: Weight (kg) ÷ Stature (cm) ÷ Stature (cm) x 10,000
or Weight (lb) ÷ Stature (in) ÷ Stature (in) x 703

Published May 30, 2000 (modified 10/16/00).
SOURCE: Developed by the National Center for Health Statistics in collaboration with
the National Center for Chronic Disease Prevention and Health Promotion (2000).
http://www.cdc.gov/growthcharts

SAFER · HEALTHIER · PEOPLE™

Girls: 2-20 Years
Stature-For-Age & Weight-For-Age Percentiles

Reprinted from the Centers for Disease Control & Prevention website, www.cdc.gov

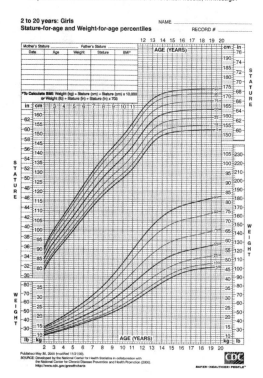

2 to 20 years: Girls
Stature-for-age and Weight-for-age percentiles

Girls: 2-20 Years
Body Mass Index-For-Age Percentiles

Reprinted from the Centers for Disease Control & Prevention website, www.cdc.gov

2 to 20 years: Girls
Body mass index-for-age percentiles

NAME _____

RECORD # _____

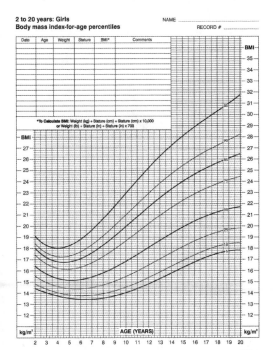

*To Calculate BMI: Weight (kg) ÷ Stature (cm) ÷ Stature (cm) x 10,000
or Weight (lb) ÷ Stature (in) ÷ Stature (in) x 703

AGE (YEARS)

Published May 30, 2000 (modified 10/16/00).
SOURCE: Developed by the National Center for Health Statistics in collaboration with
the National Center for Chronic Disease Prevention and Health Promotion (2000).
http://www.cdc.gov/growthcharts

SAFER · HEALTHIER · PEOPLE™

Boys: Weight-For-Stature Percentiles

Reprinted from Centers for Disease Control and Prevention website, www.cdc.gov

Weight-for-stature percentiles: Boys

NAME _____

RECORD # _____

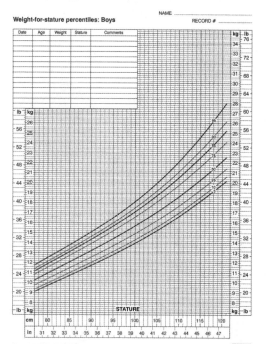

Published May 30, 2000 (modified 10/16/00).
SOURCE: Developed by the National Center for Health Statistics in collaboration with
the National Center for Chronic Disease Prevention and Health Promotion (2000).
http://www.cdc.gov/growthcharts

SAFER · HEALTHIER · PEOPLE™

Girls: Weight-For-Stature Percentiles

Reprinted from the Centers for Disease Control & Prevention website, www.cdc.gov

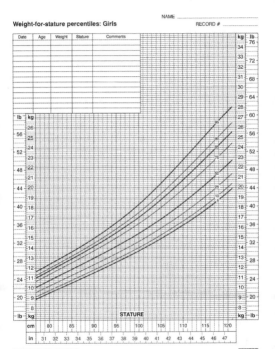

Weight-for-stature percentiles: Girls

NAME _____

RECORD # _____

Published May 30, 2000 (modified 10/16/00).

SOURCE: Developed by the National Center for Health Statistics in collaboration with
the National Center for Chronic Disease Prevention and Health Promotion (2000).
http://www.cdc.gov/growthcharts

SAFER · HEALTHIER · PEOPLE™

Index

Page left blank for notes

Page left blank for notes

Page left blank for notes

Page left blank for notes

Page left blank for notes

Page left blank for notes

Page left blank for notes

Page left blank for notes

Page left blank for notes

Page left blank for notes

Page left blank for notes

Page left blank for notes

Page left blank for notes

Page left blank for notes

Page left blank for notes

Page left blank for notes

Tarascon Publishing Order Form on Next Page

Price per Copy by Number of Copies Ordered				
Total # of each ordered →	1–9	10–49	50–99	≥100
Tarascon Pocket Pharmacopoeia				
• Classic shirt pocket edition	$11.95	$10.95	$9.95	$8.95
• Deluxe lab coat pocket edition	$19.95	$16.95	$14.95	$13.95
• PDA edition on CD, 12 month subscription	$32.95	$28.00	$26.36	$24.70
Other Tarascon Pocketbooks				
• Tarascon Pediatric Outpatient Pocketbook	$14.95	$13.45	$11.94	$10.44
• Tarascon Internal Med & Crit Care Pocketbook	$14.95	$13.45	$11.94	$10.44
• Tarascon Primary Care Pocketbook	$14.95	$13.45	$11.94	$10.44
• Tarascon Pediatric Emergency Pocketbook	$14.95	$13.45	$11.94	$10.44
• Tarascon Adult Emergency Pocketbook	$14.95	$13.45	$11.94	$10.44
• Tarascon Pocket Orthopaedica	$14.95	$13.45	$11.94	$10.44
• How to be a Truly Excellent Junior Med Student	$9.95	$8.25	$7.45	$6.95
Tarascon Rapid Reference Cards & Magnifier				
• Tarascon Quick P450 Enzyme Reference Card	$1.95	$1.85	$1.75	$1.65
• Tarascon Quick Cardiac Arrest / Emergency	$1.95	$1.85	$1.75	$1.65
• Tarascon Quick Pediatric Reference Card	$1.95	$1.85	$1.75	$1.65
• Tarascon Quick HTN/LDL Reference Card	$1.95	$1.85	$1.75	$1.65
• Tarascon Fresnel Magnifying Lens and Ruler	$1.00	$0.89	$0.78	$0.66
Other Recommended Pocketbooks				
• Managing Contraception	$10.00	$9.75	$9.50	$9.25
• OB/GYN & Infertility	$19.95	$19.55	$19.25	$18.80
• Airway Cam Pocket Guide to Intubation	$14.95	$14.55	$14.25	$13.80
• Thompson's Rheumatology Pocket Reference	$14.95	$14.55	$14.25	$13.80
• Reproductive Endocrinology/Infertility-Pocket	$14.95	$14.55	$14.25	$13.80
• Reproductive Endocrinology/Infertility-Desk	$24.95	$24.55	$24.20	$23.80

Shipping & Handling (based on subtotal on next page order form)					
If subtotal is →	≤$12	$13–29.99	$30–75.99	$76–200	$201–700
Standard shipping	$1.50	$2.75	$6.25	$8.00	$16.00
UPS 2-day air (no PO boxes)	$13.00	$15.00	$17.00	$20.00	$40.00

Tarascon Pocket Pharmacopoeia® Deluxe PDA Edition

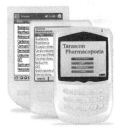

Features
- Palm / Pocket PC / BlackBerry versions
- Meticulously peer-reviewed drug information
- Multiple drug interaction checking
- Continuous internet auto-updates
- Extended memory card support
- Multiple tables & formulas
- Complete customer privacy
  Download a FREE 30-day trial version at www.tarascon.com
  Subscriptions thereafter priced at $2.50/month

Ordering Books From Tarascon Publishing

INTERNET	**MAIL**	**FAX**	**PHONE**
Order through our OnLine store with your credit card at www.tarascon.com	Mail order & check to: **Tarascon Publishing** PO Box 517 Lompoc, CA 93438	Fax credit card orders 24 hrs/day toll free to **877.929.9926**	For phone orders or customer service, call **800.929.9926**

Name	Company name (if applicable)
Address	

City	State	Zip	Residential ☐ Business ☐
Phone		Email	

TARASCON POCKET PHARMACOPOEIA®	Quantity	Price*
Classic Shirt-Pocket Edition		$
Deluxe Labcoat Pocket Edition		$
PDA software on CD-ROM, 12 month subscription‡		$
OTHER TARASCON POCKETBOOKS		
Tarascon Pediatric Outpatient Pocketbook		$
Tarascon Internal Medicine & Critical Care Pocketbook		$
Tarascon Primary Care Pocketbook		$
Tarascon Pediatric Emergency Pocketbook		$
Tarascon Adult Emergency Pocketbook		$
Tarascon Pocket Orthopaedica®		$
How to be a Truly Excellent Junior Medical Student		$
TARASCON RAPID REFERENCE CARDS & MAGNIFIER		
Tarascon Quick P450 Enzyme Reference Card		$
Tarascon Quick Cardiac Arrest / Emergency Card		$
Tarascon Quick Pediatric Reference Card		$
Tarascon Quick HTN & LDL Reference Card		$
Tarascon Fresnel Magnifying Lens and Ruler		$
OTHER RECOMMENDED POCKETBOOKS		
Managing Contraception		$
OB/GYN & Infertility		$
Airway Cam Pocket Guide to Intubation		$
Thompson's Rheumatology Pocket Reference		$
Reproductive Endocrinology/Infertility Pocket edition		$
Reproductive Endocrinology/Infertility Desk edition		$

*See prior page for prices / shipping. ‡Or download today at www.tarascon.com

☐ VISA ☐ Mastercard ☐ American Express ☐ Discover		**Subtotal**	$
Card number		CA only add 7.25% sales tax	$
Exp date	CID code number	Shipping / handling*	$
Signature		**TOTAL**	$